CyberMedics

CyberMedics: Navigating AI and Security in the Medical Field is a comprehensive exploration of the transformative role of artificial intelligence (AI) in healthcare and the critical importance of securing medical data in an increasingly digital world. As AI technologies revolutionize diagnostics, treatment planning, and patient care, they also introduce new challenges related to data privacy, ethical considerations, and cybersecurity.

This book offers a balanced perspective, providing healthcare professionals, technologists, and policymakers with the tools they need to understand and navigate the intersection of AI and security. Through detailed case studies, expert insights, and practical guidance, readers will discover how AI can be leveraged to improve patient outcomes while maintaining the highest standards of data protection.

Key topics include:

- AI in healthcare, exploring how emerging technologies like machine learning, natural language processing, and predictive analytics are poised to reshape the industry
- the ethical implications of AI in healthcare
- strategies for safeguarding sensitive information against cyber threats
- future frameworks governing the use of AI in medical settings

Whether you're on the front lines of patient care, involved in healthcare IT, or shaping policy, *CyberMedics: Navigating AI and Security in the Medical Field* equips you with the knowledge to make informed decisions in a rapidly evolving landscape, ensuring that innovation and security go hand in hand to enhance the quality of care.

CyberMedics

Navigating AI and Security in the Medical Field

Edited by
Varun Sapra, Rohit Tanwar, and Luxmi Sapra

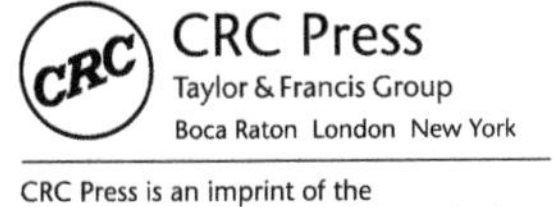

CRC Press
Taylor & Francis Group
Boca Raton London New York

CRC Press is an imprint of the
Taylor & Francis Group, an **informa** business

Designed cover image: ©Shutterstock

First edition published 2025
by CRC Press
2385 NW Executive Center Drive, Suite 320, Boca Raton FL 33431

and by CRC Press
4 Park Square, Milton Park, Abingdon, Oxon, OX14 4RN

CRC Press is an imprint of Taylor & Francis Group, LLC

© 2025 selection and editorial matter, Varun Sapra, Rohit Tanwar, and Luxmi Sapra; individual chapters, the contributors

ISBN: 9781032847023 (hbk)
ISBN: 9781032854182 (pbk)
ISBN: 9781003518075 (ebk)

DOI: 10.1201/9781003518075

Typeset in Sabon
by Newgen Publishing UK

Contents

About the editors

Varun Sapra is currently Associate Professor with the School of Computer Science, University of Petroleum and Energy Studies, Dehradun, India. He is an accomplished academic professional with 18 years of experience in both academia and industry. Holding a Ph.D. in Computer Science, he brings a wealth of expertise to his teaching and research endeavors. He has to his credit more than 40 research papers in peer-reviewed international journals and conferences, two patents granted and several copyrights and edited books, including chapters in international journals and publishers.

Rohit Tanwar received his bachelor's degree (B.Tech) in CSE from Kurukshetra University, Kurukshetra, India, and master's degree (M.Tech) in CSE from YMCA University of Science and Technology, Faridabad, India. Dr. Tanwar was awarded his Ph.D. in the year 2019 from Kurukshetra University. He has more than 13 years of experience in teaching. Currently, he works as Associate Professor in the School of Computer Science and Engineering, Shri Mata Vaishno Devi University, Katra. His areas of interest include Network Security, Optimization Techniques, Internet of Things, Healthcare, Wireless Sensor Networks, etc. He has been associated with many conferences throughout India as TPC member and session chair.

Dr. Tanwar has published more than 50 research papers in different journals of international repute. He has seven books and six patents to his credit. He is a senior IEEE member and Senior EAI member. He is also listed as editorial board review member in different SCI and Scopus Indexed Journals. Dr. Tanwar supervises many postgraduate and Ph.D. students in the field of network security. He is an active reviewer of various projects that are submitted to UGC for funding.

Luxmi Sapra is Associate Professor at Graphic Era Hill University, Dehradun, India. She has done her Doctorate in Computer Science and Engineering from NorthCap University and received her Masters in Technology from MDU, Rohtak, India. She has approximately 18 years of research and teaching experience. She has to her credit more than 40 publications in reputed journals and conferences including Elsevier, Springer, and IEEE. She is also a reviewer of various international journals. She received 3AI Pinnacle Award for Women in AI and Analytics in 2020. She was also awarded 4th Himalaya Nari Shakti Samman-2022 on the occasion of Women's Day 8th March 2022 at DIT University, Dehradun. Her research areas include Cyber Security, Machine Learning, Artificial Intelligence and Healthcare. She has published five patents and chaired sessions in international conferences.

Contributors

Ambika Aggarwal
Associate Professor, UPES, India

Shahina Anwarul
Assistant Professor, UPES, India

Ashutosh Bhatt
Associate Professor, Swami Rama Himalayan University, India

Prachi Chhabra
Assistant Professor, Academy of Technical Education, India

Anubhav Dubey
Assistant Professor, Maharana Pratap College of Pharmacy, India

Srimathi Elango
Student, Kongu Engineering College, India

Rekha Handa
Assistant Professor, Guru Nanak Dev University, India

Amandeep Singh Kalra
Professor, Dept of Computer Science and Engineering, Gulzar Group of
Institutions, India

Samyuktha Kathirvel
Student, Kongu Engineering College, India

Randeep Kaur
Assistant Professor, Khalsa College, Amritsar, India

Neha Kaushal
Assistant Professor, Gulzar Group of Institutions, India

Bhawna Kaushik
Assistant Professor, Smt. Sushma Swaraj Govt. College for Girls, Ballabgarh, Faridabad, India

Sunil Kumar
Assistant Professor, CSJM University, India

Mamta Kumari
Assistant Professor, Maharana Pratap College of Pharmacy, India

Ramnayan Mishra
Assistant Professor, CSJM University, India

Abinaya Nagarajan
Assistant Professor, Hindusthan Institute of Technology, India

Jayadharshini Periasamy
Assistant Professor, Kongu Engineering College, India

Santhiya Saminathan
Assistant Professor, Kongu Engineering College, India

Rashid Rafiq Shah
Assistant Professor, Gulzar Group of Institutions, India

Honey Sharma
Professor and Campus Director, Dept. of Computer Science and Engineering, Gulzar Group of Institutions, India

Nipun Sharma
Assistant Professor, Dept. of Computer Science and Engineering, Gulzar Group of Institutions, India

Roohi Sille
Assistant Professor, UPES, India

Prabal Pratap Singh
Assistant Professor, CSJM University, India

Sonal Talreja
Assistant Professor, UPES, India

Abirami Thiyagarajan
Associate Professor, Kongu Engineering College, India

Chapter 1

Enhancing energy efficiency and safety in smart homes

A framework for secure IoT-driven home automation with facial recognition and sensor networks

Shahina Anwarul

1.1 INTRODUCTION

The expansion in the prominence of IoT has spread to different domains like intelligent parking systems, savvy homes, smart gadgets, etc. [1–3]. The execution of IoT in homes is for energy observation and conservation while accomplishing and keeping up with specific comfort levels. SHAS utilizing IoT comprises three significant parts as displayed in Figure 1.1 [4]. The house with sensors and network comprises different sensors that are deployed to gather data. It contains the different sensors and actuators which are in correspondence with the microcontroller like Raspberry Pi. The information is conveyed over the Wi-Fi network by the microcontroller and is put away in the Cloud. The information from the Cloud is shown on the application and the client provides the necessary command in view of which a predefined move is made by the microcontroller. The actuators then, at that point, act in view of the information got by them.

Home automation can be characterized as the robotization of normal routine household exercises while having essential control over the devices. The facial recognition technology helps to create a more intelligent and energy-efficient smart home by enabling personalized and efficient energy management [5]. Facial recognition technology can also be used to detect the presence of occupants in different rooms of the home, allowing for more precise and efficient control of the energy systems [6]. For example, the system can turn off the lights and adjust the temperature in rooms that are unoccupied, reducing unnecessary energy consumption [7]. Face identification is done by the analysis and comparison of essential facial features and expressions. It is a technology that aims to make our world more intelligent and safe. It can be used for verification as well as recognition of an individual. Home automation means using technology to control everyday household activities automatically while having basic control over devices. Here are a few reasons why we need home automation:

DOI: 10.1201/9781003518075-1

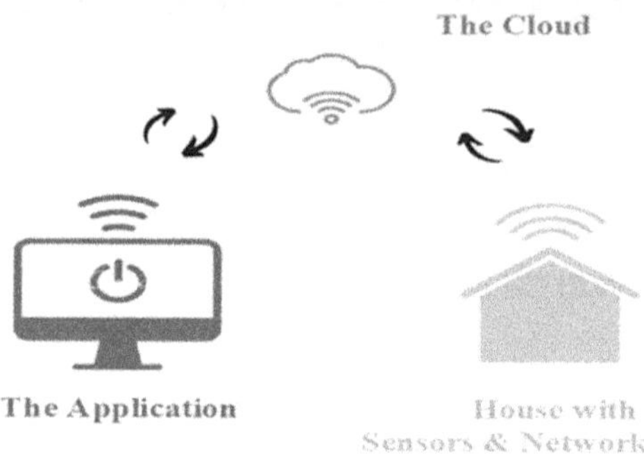

Figure 1.1 The architecture of the SHAS.

> *Improved Safety:* This is a major reason people want to automate their homes. Sensors like PIR (passive infrared) can collect data and communicate with devices to perform simple tasks like opening doors and turning lights on and off. Using a smart app, other electrical appliances like heaters, washing machines, and refrigerators can also be controlled.
>
> *Convenient Lighting:* Home automation can control pathway lighting based on movement. It can also alert users to any suspicious activity.
>
> *Time-Saving and Peace of Mind:* Automating these complex tasks creates an environment that the user can easily control and monitor. It saves a lot of time and provides a sense of security, allowing users to perform tasks with just a tap on their device, even if they initially forget to do so.

When we talk about these features, the complexity and cost of setting up and maintaining such a large system can be high. Therefore, we need to implement a proper and precise system that is easy for everyone in the house to use, so they can interact with it even when away from home. To address this, an energy efficient framework for smart home automation system is proposed in the chapter.

1.2 CHALLENGES AND PROPOSED SOLUTIONS IN SMART HOME AUTOMATION SYSTEMS

Smart home automation systems offer significant advantages in terms of convenience, energy efficiency, and security. However, they also present several challenges that must be addressed to ensure effective implementation and operation. Here are some detailed challenges associated with smart home automation systems [8–10]:

1.2.1 Interoperability and compatibility

One of the primary challenges is ensuring that various devices and systems from different manufacturers can communicate and work together seamlessly. The lack of standardization across devices often leads to compatibility issues. Different protocols (e.g., Zigbee, Z-Wave, Wi-Fi) may not always be compatible, complicating the integration process. The suggested solutions to overcome this challenge are [11]:

- Standardization: Promote and adopt industry standards like Matter, which aims to improve interoperability across different manufacturers' devices.
- Unified Hubs: Develop and use smart home hubs that can bridge various communication protocols (e.g., Zigbee, Z-Wave, Wi-Fi) to ensure compatibility among devices.
- Open APIs: Encourage manufacturers to provide open APIs, allowing third-party developers to create integration solutions.

1.2.2 Security and privacy

Smart home systems are vulnerable to cyber-attacks, which can compromise personal data and home security. Ensuring robust encryption, secure authentication mechanisms, and regular updates to address vulnerabilities are critical. Privacy concerns also arise as these systems often collect and store large amounts of personal data, necessitating strict data protection measures. The proposed solutions to address this challenge are [12]:

- Strong Encryption: Implement end-to-end encryption for data transmitted between devices and to the Cloud.
- Regular Updates: Ensure devices receive regular firmware and software updates to patch vulnerabilities.
- Two-Factor Authentication (2FA): Use 2FA to add an extra layer of security for accessing smart home systems.
- Privacy Policies: Develop and enforce strict privacy policies to protect user data and ensure compliance with regulations like GDPR.

1.2.3 Complexity and usability

The complexity of installing and configuring smart home devices can be a barrier for many users. Ensuring that these systems are user-friendly and accessible to non-technical users is essential. Designing intuitive user interfaces and providing comprehensive customer support can help mitigate this challenge. The suggested solutions to overcome these challenges are [13]:

- User-Friendly Interfaces: Design intuitive user interfaces with simple, clear instructions and easy-to-navigate menus.
- Automated Setup: Implement automated setup processes to minimize user effort in configuring devices.
- Comprehensive Support: Provide robust customer support, including detailed manuals, online resources, and responsive help desks.

1.2.4 Reliability and dependability

The reliability of smart home systems is crucial, especially when they are used for critical functions such as security or health monitoring. Devices and systems must be dependable and able to operate without frequent failures or downtime. This requires high-quality hardware, robust software, and reliable internet connectivity. The suggested solutions to overcome this issue are [13]:

- High-Quality Components: Use high-quality hardware components to enhance device reliability.
- Redundancy: Implement redundant systems and backup power supplies to ensure continuous operation during outages.
- Regular Maintenance: Schedule regular maintenance checks and updates to keep systems running smoothly.

1.2.5 Cost and affordability

The initial cost of smart home devices and the ongoing expenses for maintenance, subscription services, and potential upgrades can be significant. Making these technologies more affordable is necessary to drive widespread adoption, especially among average consumers [14].

- Affordable Options: Develop a range of products at various price points to cater to different budgets.
- Incentives and Subsidies: Governments and utilities can offer incentives or subsidies to reduce the cost burden on consumers.
- Bundle Offers: Provide bundled packages of smart devices at discounted rates.

1.2.6 Energy management and efficiency

While smart home systems are designed to improve energy efficiency, achieving this in practice can be challenging. Effective energy management requires precise control and coordination among various devices. Additionally, educating users on how to maximize energy savings through proper use of the system is important. The discussed issue can be resolved by considering these suggested solutions [15].

- Smart Algorithms: Use machine learning algorithms to optimize energy consumption based on usage patterns.
- User Education: Educate users on how to use smart home systems effectively to maximize energy savings.
- Real-Time Monitoring: Provide real-time energy consumption data to help users make informed decisions about their energy use.

1.2.7 Scalability

As users add more devices to their smart home ecosystem, ensuring that the system can scale effectively without degrading performance is crucial. Scalability issues can arise from limited network bandwidth, insufficient processing power, or inadequate storage capabilities and the suggested solutions to overcome these issues are [16]:

- Robust Network Infrastructure: Ensure that home networks are capable of handling increased traffic from multiple devices by using advanced routers and network extenders.
- Cloud Services: Leverage cloud computing for processing and storing large amounts of data, reducing the load on local systems.

1.2.8 Environmental concerns

The production, use, and disposal of smart home devices raise environmental concerns. These devices often contain materials that are difficult to recycle, and their energy consumption during use contributes to their overall environmental footprint. Developing more sustainable products and encouraging responsible disposal practices are important considerations [17].

- Sustainable Materials: Use environmentally friendly materials in the production of smart home devices.
- Recycling Programs: Implement recycling programs to properly dispose of and recycle old devices.
- Energy-Efficient Devices: Design devices that are energy-efficient and have a low environmental impact. ·

1.2.9 Dependence on internet connectivity

Many smart home systems rely heavily on internet connectivity to function properly. Any disruption in internet service can render these systems ineffective, posing a significant challenge, especially in areas with unreliable or limited internet access. These issues can be resolved by the following solutions [16].

- Local Control Options: Ensure that devices can function locally without internet connectivity for essential operations.
- Offline Capabilities: Develop offline capabilities and local storage for critical data to maintain functionality during internet outages.

By addressing these challenges through a combination of technological advancements, regulatory measures, and user-focused solutions, the smart home industry can create more reliable, secure, and user-friendly automation systems that meet the needs of a diverse range of consumers.

1.3 THE PROPOSED SMART HOME AUTOMATION FRAMEWORK

In this section, a four-layered architecture for automating Smart Homes, as illustrated in Figure 1.2 is proposed. The framework for smart homes based on this architecture is depicted in Figure 1.3. Here's how it works:

Camera Module and Facial Recognition: The camera module captures live face images using integrated sensors and a Facial Recognition System (FRS). Users create a database of authorized occupants, and upon entry, the subject's face is recorded and compared to the registered database. If there's a match, home appliances are activated. We use Multi-Task Cascaded Convolutional Networks (MTCNN) [18] for face detection and Hybrid Ensemble Convolutional Neural Network (HE-CNN) [19] for recognition. If there's no match, the homeowner is alerted via registered contact numbers and email IDs.

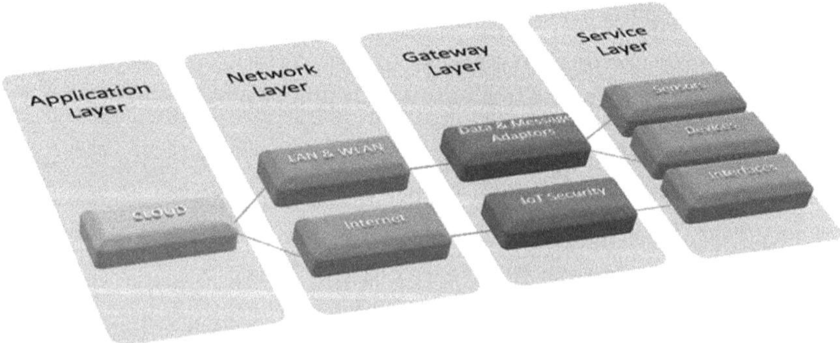

Figure 1.2 A demonstration of four-layered IoT architecture for home automation systems.

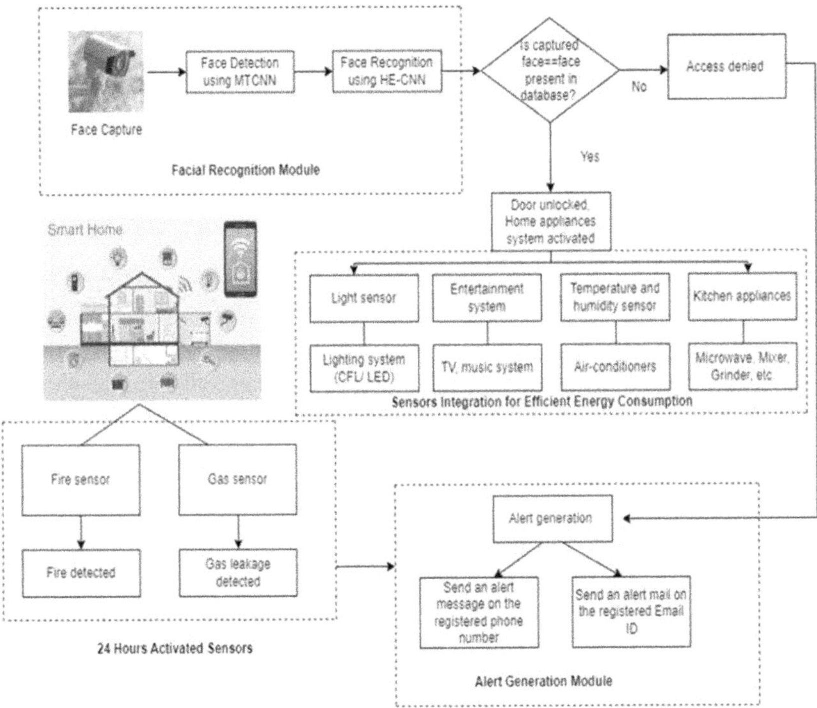

Figure 1.3 The framework for smart home automation.

Safety Measures: To prevent accidents like fires or gas leaks, all home appliances are instantly turned off, and the sprinkler system activates in case of a fire. Appliances are also shut off and occupants alerted if current dissipation exceeds threshold values.

Service Layer: This layer consists of various sensors and actuators communicating over a framework to the Cloud/Internet. These sensors act as services, transforming cultural artifacts into smart services. The data collected by this layer is crucial for individual home smartness and influences modern communication equipment. It plays a key role in creating a data-driven IoT model.

Gateway Layer: This layer ensures the secure communication of gathered information to higher layers. It handles the security aspects of IoT frameworks and ensures the integrity of sensitive data transmitted from sensors to upper layers.

Network Layer: Responsible for identifying various protocols used in IoT systems.

Application/Cloud Layer: Deals with model training and cloud architecture implementation. Overall, this architecture enhances the

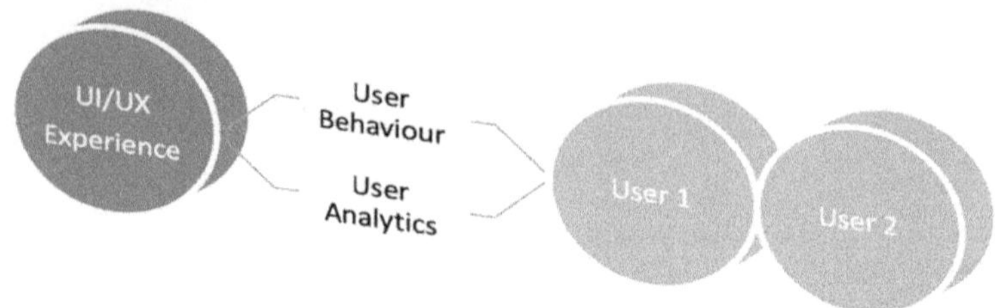

Figure 1.4 Bridging the UI gap in IoT systems.

convenience and safety of Smart Homes, allowing users to interact with the system seamlessly through their own devices and ensuring secure communication and data handling throughout the system.

1.4. DISCUSSION ON THE NEED OF INTERACTIVE USER INTERFACE (UI) FOR SMART HOME AUTOMATION

After investigating various strategies for IoT-based smart home automation systems, a notable gap in the development of a user interface specific to HAS (Home Automation System) is identified. It became evident that there is a universal need for an engaging and user-friendly interface to operate these applications effectively. Consequently, there is an urgent demand for interactive user interfaces tailored to automated systems. Figure 1.4 illustrates the research gap concerning the creation of UI in IoT Systems.

In order to enhance the user experience and optimize IoT user interfaces for household appliances, it is essential to analyze user history, sessions, behavior, and other pertinent factors. For instance, consider a household where two children, aged 10, along with a working father, a full-time house-wife, and grandparents are users of the same smart-home IoT system. Each user group has unique requirements, challenges, and relationships, influencing their interactions with the applications and UI. For instance, working mothers may seek to minimize time spent on household tasks and thus may interact with the system less frequently. Nonetheless, the dashboard or application must remain user-friendly for smooth engagement when users do interact with the UI. Table 1.1 delineates these interactions, objectives, and behaviors, along with relevant UI attributes for each user group.

1.5 CONCLUSION AND FUTURE SCOPE

The integration of energy-efficient technologies in smart homes, facilitated by IoT, Machine Learning, and Cloud services, significantly enhances the quality of life both at home and in the workplace. This chapter has proposed

Table 1.1 User interactions and attributes to be taken care while building a UI

User Category	User Behavior	User Purpose to Interact	UI Attributes to be Taken Care
Limited users (House makers, Grand-parents)	These are the users who interact with the system only for certain purposes and they use repeatedly the same thing over a time period.	• On/Off appliances • Door lock/unlock • Any video interactions	• Clear understanding of UI/UX • Ease access of the system/features
Intermediate users (Children and Adults)	These are the users who interact with the system for trying out new things and exploring the features and also like to make the surroundings smart.	• Control smartly using assistants • Checking analytics • Assisting limited users	• Modular to add/ remove services • Ease in analyzing the system
Market users (Creators/ Buyers)	These are the active users who are involved most of the time with the system so that they can make and enjoy most out of the implemented system.	• Assisting limited, intermediate users • Analyzing and implementing features for above users.	• Checking the requirements of the above users and implementing the system. • While giving upgrades, consider the behavior of limited users.

a comprehensive framework for a Smart Home Automation System (SHAS) that incorporates a Facial Recognition System (FRS) and an integrated network of sensors. The FRS improves the accuracy and effectiveness of energy system regulation by detecting residents' locations within the home. The sensor network, including gas, fire, light, temperature, and humidity sensors, ensures safety and optimizes energy consumption. Additionally, the design and implementation of an intuitive user interface have been discussed, emphasizing the importance of user-friendly interactions with the smart home system.

Future research in smart home automation should focus on developing universal interoperability standards to ensure seamless device integration, implementing advanced security protocols to protect against cyber threats, and enhancing user interfaces to be more intuitive and accessible. Additionally, leveraging sophisticated AI and Machine Learning algorithms can better predict user behavior and automate tasks more efficiently. Emphasizing sustainable solutions by using eco-friendly materials and energy-efficient technologies will reduce environmental impact. Ensuring scalability and flexibility will allow smart home systems to adapt to emerging technologies and innovations, ultimately providing greater convenience, efficiency, and security for users. The deployment of the proposed framework for the smart home automation can also be done.

REFERENCES

[1] C. Stolojescu-Crisan, C. Crisan, & B. P. Butunoi, "An IoT-based smart home automation system," *Sensors*, 21(11), 3784, 2021.

[2] A. Aditya, S. Anwarul, R. Tanwar, & S. K. V. Koneru, "An IoT assisted intelligent parking system (IPS) for smart cities," *Procedia Computer Science*, 218, 1045–1054, 2023.

[3] P. Chithaluru, S. Kumar, A. Singh, A. Benslimane, & S. K. Jangir, "An Energy-efficient routing scheduling based on Fuzzy ranking scheme for internet of things," *IEEE Internet of Things Journal*, 9(10), 7251–7260, 2021.

[4] U. Pujari, D. Patil, D. Bahadure, & M. Asnodkar, "Internet of things based integrated smart home automation system," In *2nd International Conference on Communication & Information Processing (ICCIP)*, 2020.

[5] M. Alilou, B. Tousi, & H. Shayeghi, "Home energy management in a residential smart micro grid under stochastic penetration of solar panels and electric vehicles," *Solar Energy*, 212, 6–18, 2020.

[6] S. Anwarul, & S. Dahiya, "Rectified DenseNet169-based automated criminal recognition system for the prediction of crime prone areas using face recognition," *Journal of Electronic Imaging*, 31(4), 043055–043055, 2022.

[7] Y. Kortli, M. Jridi, A. Al Falou, & M. Atri, "Face recognition systems: A survey," *Sensors*, 20(2), 342, 2020.

[8] B. L. R. Stojkoska, & K. V. Trivodaliev, "A review of Internet of Things for smart home: Challenges and solutions," *Journal of Cleaner Production*, 140, 1454–1464, 2017.

[9] N. G. Vasilescu, P. Pocatilu, & M. Doinea, "IoT security challenges for smart homes," In *Education, Research and Business Technologies: Proceedings of 21st International Conference on Informatics in Economy (IE 2022)* (pp. 41–49). Singapore: Springer Nature Singapore, 2023.

[10] I. Malik, A. Bhardwaj, H. Bhardwaj, & A. Sakalle, "IoT-enabled smart homes: Architecture, challenges, and issues," In Divya Upadhyay Mishra & Shanu Sharma (eds.), *Revolutionizing Industrial Automation through the Convergence of Artificial Intelligence and the Internet of Things* (pp. 160–176). IGI Global, 2023.

[11] M. C. Marin, M. Cerutti, S. Batista, & M. Brambilla, "A multi-protocol IoT platform for enhanced interoperability and standardization in smart home," In *2024 IEEE 21st Consumer Communications & Networking Conference (CCNC)* (pp. 1–6). IEEE, 2024.

[12] A. Aldahmani, B. Ouni, T. Lestable, & M. Debbah, "Cyber-security of embedded IoTs in smart homes: Challenges, requirements, countermeasures, and trends," *IEEE Open Journal of Vehicular Technology*, 4, 281–292, 2023.

[13] E. Becks, P. Zdankin, V. Matkovic, & T. Weis, "Complexity of smart home setups: a qualitative user study on smart home assistance and implications on technical requirements," *Technologies*, 11(1), 9, 2023.

[14] B. Akhmetzhanov, B. Akhmetzhanov, S. Ozdemir, & N. Zhakiyev, "Advancing affordable IoT solutions in smart homes to enhance independence and autonomy of the elderly," *Journal of Infrastructure, Policy and Development*, 8(3), 2899, 2024.

[15] B. Han, Y. Zahraoui, M. Mubin, S. Mekhilef, M. Seyedmahmoudian, & A. Stojcevski, "Home energy management systems: a review of the concept, architecture, and scheduling strategies," *IEEE Access*, 11, 19999–20025, 2023.

[16] A. Dhar Dwivedi, R. Singh, K. Kaushik, R. Rao Mukkamala, & W. S. Alnumay, "Blockchain and artificial intelligence for 5G-enabled Internet of Things: Challenges, opportunities, and solutions," *Transactions on Emerging Telecommunications Technologies*, 35(4), e4329, 2024.

[17] M. Ehsanifar, F. Dekamini, C. Spulbar, R. Birau, M. Khazaei, & I. C. Bărbăcioru, "A sustainable pattern of waste management and energy efficiency in smart homes using the internet of things (IoT)," *Sustainability*, 15(6), 5081, 2023.

[18] K. Zhang, Z. Zhang, Z. Li, & Y. Qiao, "Joint face detection and alignment using multitask cascaded convolutional networks," *IEEE Signal Processing Letters*, 23(10), 1499–1503, 2016.

[19] S. Anwarul, T. Choudhury, & S. Dahiya, "A novel hybrid ensemble convolutional neural network for face recognition by optimizing hyperparameters," *Nonlinear Engineering*, 12(1), 20220290, 2023.

Chapter 2

Embracing the future

Tracing the role of Artificial Intelligence (AI) and Internet of Things (IoT) in secure agricultural automation

Shahina Anwarul

2.1 INTRODUCTION

Agriculture, often hailed as the backbone of any nation, stands as a corner-stone for economic growth and food security [1]. Farming has always been crucial for societies everywhere. It's been around for thousands of years and has shaped how civilizations grow and take care of people. Agriculture, which is all about growing crops and raising animals, shows how strong and creative humans can be. It's like a part of who we are, always changing and finding new ways to thrive in our world. Traditionally, farming has been a labor-intensive endeavor, with farmers relying on manual labor and continuous monitoring to cultivate the land and produce food. For centuries, generations of farmers have toiled under the sun, tilling the soil, sowing seeds, and reaping the harvests that sustain communities and nations. This intimate connection between humans and the land has been the essence of agriculture, shaping cultures, traditions, and livelihoods across the globe.

However, the agricultural landscape is undergoing a profound trans-formation, fueled by rapid advancements in technology and the onset of the Fourth Industrial Revolution, often referred to as "Industry 4.0." This technological revolution, marked by the integration of digital, physical, and biological systems, is transforming various industries and societies, agriculture included [2]. At the heart of this transformation lies the integration of cutting-edge technologies such as the Internet of Things (IoT), Deep Learning (DL), Cloud Computing, and Computer Vision [3–6]. These technologies are revolutionizing every aspect of agricultural operations, from planting and irrigation to harvesting and distribution. The convergence of digital innovations with traditional farming practices has given rise to "Smart and Sustainable Agriculture" systems, heralding a new era of farming efficiency, productivity, and sustainability.

The traditional methodologies of agriculture, reliant on constant supervi-sion and manual intervention, are being supplanted by automated systems that offer precise and real-time monitoring and management of agricultural activities. Gone are the days of labor-intensive farming, where farmers had

DOI: 10.1201/9781003518075-2

to rely on their instincts and experience to navigate the uncertainties of weather, pests, and crop diseases. With the advent of smart agriculture systems, these challenges are being addressed with unprecedented efficiency and accuracy [7]. The deployment of IoT sensors enables farmers to gather real-time data on soil moisture, air quality, weather conditions, and crop health, empowering them to make informed decisions and optimize resource allocation [8]. Deep Learning algorithms scrutinize extensive datasets to discern patterns, predict outcomes, and optimize crop yields [9]. Cloud Computing provides a scalable and secure platform for data storage, processing, and analysis, enabling seamless collaboration and decision-making across agricultural ecosystems [10]. Computer Vision technologies streamline tasks like pest detection, weed identification, and crop monitoring, thereby decreasing reliance on manual labor and mitigating human error [11].

This shift towards automation in agriculture is not merely a passing trend but a necessary evolution to meet the increasing global food demands efficiently and sustainably. With the world's population projected to approach nearly ten billion by 2050, the pressure on agricultural systems to produce more food with fewer resources is intensifying. Climate change, resource scarcity, and environmental degradation further exacerbate these challenges, underscoring the urgency of adopting innovative solutions to ensure food security for future generations. Smart and Sustainable Agriculture systems offer a pathway towards achieving this goal, by leveraging technology to boost productivity, optimize resource utilization, and reduce environmental impact [12]. By embracing automation, farmers can increase yields, reduce costs, and mitigate risks, ensuring the long-term viability of agricultural operations in an increasingly uncertain world. The incorporation of IoT and Artificial Intelligence technologies into agriculture signifies a fundamental change in how we farm the land and nourish the world. By leveraging digital innovations, farmers can transform traditional farming practices into smart, sustainable, and resilient agricultural systems that meet the challenges of the twenty-first century. As we embrace the future of agriculture, let us continue to harness the power of technology to nourish our communities, protect our planet, and construct a future that is more sustainable for everyone.

2.1.1 Overview of the chapter

This chapter aims to provide a comprehensive analysis of the latest technologies and approaches in smart and sustainable agriculture. It explores various strategies for agricultural automation and compares the performance of different techniques. The chapter is structured as follows:

Section 2.2: Reviews the use of Computer Vision, IoT, Cloud Computing, and Robotics in agricultural automation.

Section 2.3: In this section, a framework for agricultural automation using AI and IoT is introduced and comparison of the proposed framework with existing literature is also done to demonstrate the efficacy of our work.

Section 2.4: Highlights the importance of agricultural automation.

Section 2.5: Discusses the research gaps and challenges in smart agriculture.

Section 2.6: Concludes with future prospects and potential development directions in this field.

The following chapter will delve deeper into each of these technologies, presenting case studies, research findings, and practical applications in the agricultural sector. The objective is to offer a comprehensive insight into how smart and sustainable agriculture can transform farming methods and bolster global food security.

2.2 THE ROLE OF AUTOMATION IN AGRICULTURE

Agricultural automation entails employing advanced technologies to carry out farming activities with minimal human intervention. This includes the utilization of IoT-based systems, computer vision, robotics, and machine learning to monitor and manage various aspects of farming and the summary of these systems in existing literature is given in Table 2.1. The goal is to enhance productivity, reduce labor costs, and ensure better quality and yield of crops.

2.2.1 Internet of Things (IoT)

IoT technology facilitates the interconnection of diverse devices and sensors via the internet, enabling real-time data collection and remote monitoring, as depicted in Figure 2.1. In agriculture, IoT devices can be used to monitor soil moisture, weather conditions, crop health, and more. Subsequently, this data can undergo analysis to enable informed decision-making regarding irrigation, fertilization, and pest control, thus optimizing resource utilization and enhancing crop yield [13–16].

2.2.2 Artificial Intelligence, Computer Vision, and Deep Learning

The application of Artificial Intelligence (AI) and Computer Vision (CV) in agricultural and food processing is detailed in Figure 2.2. Computer vision, combined with deep learning, allows for the automated analysis of images captured from fields. This technology can be used for tasks such as pest detection, weed identification, crop quality assessment, and yield prediction. By employing high-resolution cameras and advanced image processing

Table 2.1 Summary of the existing literature for agricultural automation using cutting-edge technologies

Author and Year	Technology	Application Area	Methodology Used	Results
Kumar et al., 2019 [27]	AI and Computer Vision	Yield Prediction	K-Nearest Neighbors (KNN), Support Vector Machine (SVM), and Random Forest (RF)	The crop yield prediction accuracy using SVM is 72.8643%, KNN is 80.9045%, and RF is 95.8543%
Mahore et al., 2021 [28]	AI and Computer Vision	Pest Control	Masked phone estimate and masked rotation estimate image processing techniques	The injury estimation is 95%
Dorman et al., 2021 [29]	AI and Computer Vision	Plant Species Recognition	Multilayer Perceptron with Adaboosting and feature extraction is done using morphological features	The achieved precision rate is 95.42%
Roopaei et al., 2017 [30]	IoT and Cloud	Automated irrigation	Thermal imaging and Cloud of Things (CoT)	A thermal image with both low- and high-temperature values for the Irrigation Temperature Distribution Measurement (ITDM) results in a better irrigation system.
Namani et al., 2020 [31]	IoT and Cloud	Sustainable and smart agriculture	Smart drone using IoT and Cloud Computing technology	Utilization of IoT provides the cutting-edge technology in agriculture and farming for high-quality crop manufacture and benefits of public cloud in agriculture are discussed to boost sharing of resources and data storage in cost effective way.

(continued)

Table 2.1 (Cont.)

Author and Year	Technology	Application Area	Methodology Used	Results
Raghuvanshi et al., 2021 [32]	IoT and Cloud	Analysis of soil quality and the movement of animals.	Arduino, Breadboard, and sensors	This low-cost model might help farmers in utilizing lesser amount of water to grow a crop, as well as in amplifying the yields and the quality of the crops by better management of soil during crucial stages of the growth of the plant.
Ge et al., 2019 [33]	Robotics	Detection and recognition of ripe and unripe strawberries	Mask Recurrent Convolutional Neural Network (R-CNN) is used for strawberry detection	The average detection accuracy rate of ripe strawberry is 90% and unripe strawberry is 72%
Hussain et al., 2020 [34]	Robotics	Weed detection, drip irrigation, weed elimination for the wheat field	Convolutional Neural Network (CNN), 12V DC motor, NEMA 17 stepper motor, pH sensor	The precision, recall, and accuracy for weed detection is 94.7%, 92.3%, and 92.4%, respectively
Kumar et al., 2021 [35]	Robotics	Seed sowing	IoT module, seed discharger unit, ultrasonic sensors	Achieved seedling rates for different seeds such as 10 sec/2ft for groundnut, 8 sec/2ft for corn seeds, 15 sec/2ft for red gram dal, 36 sec/2ft for sesame seeds, 26 sec/2ft for almond

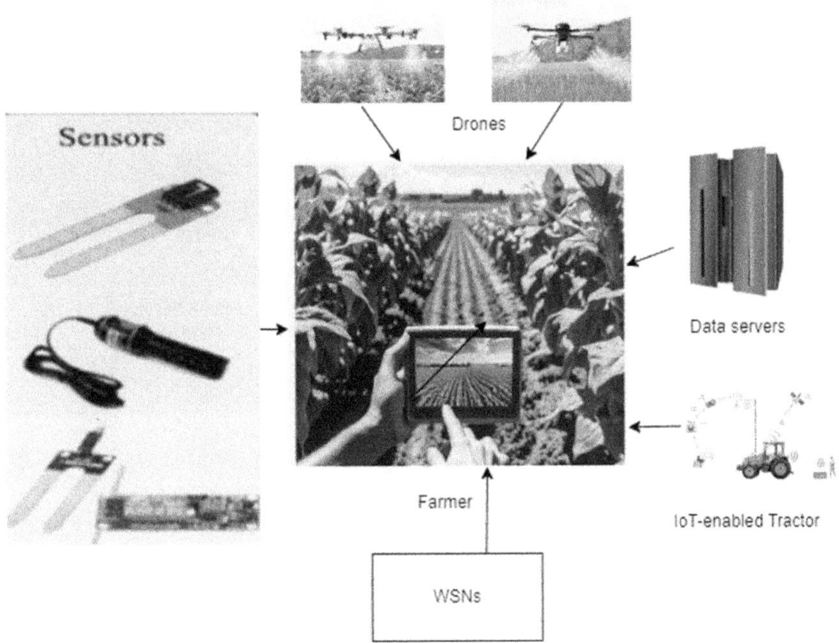

Figure 2.1 Application of IoT in agriculture automation.

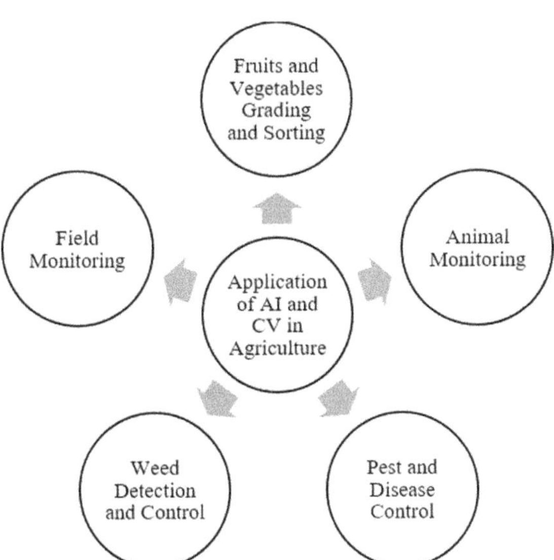

Figure 2.2 Application of AI and CV in agriculture automation.

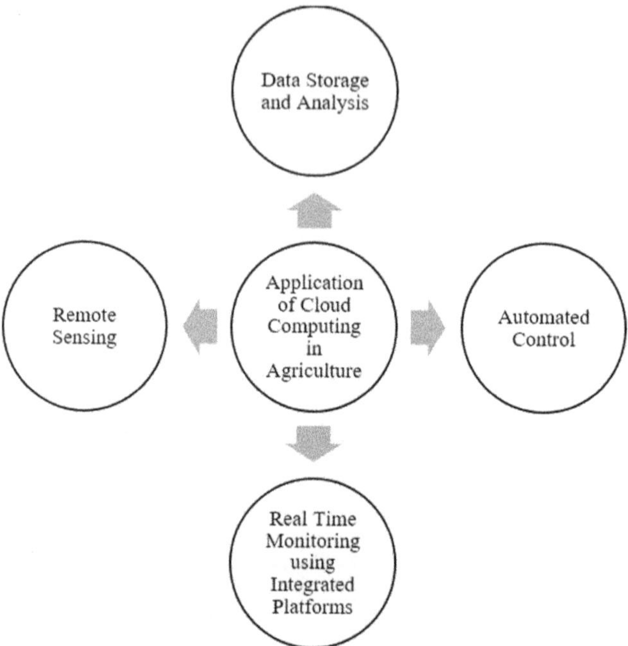

Figure 2.3 Application of cloud computing in agriculture automation.

algorithms, farmers can gain detailed insights into their crops' health and take timely actions to address any issues [17–21].

2.2.3 Cloud computing

Cloud computing provides a scalable and flexible platform for storing and processing vast amounts of agricultural data as illustrated in Figure 2.3. It enables the integration of data from various sources, including IoT sensors, drones, and satellite imagery, and allows for the deployment of sophisticated analytics and machine learning models [22]. This results in better decision-making and improved efficiency in farming operations. Cambra et al. [23] suggested an irrigation monitoring and controlling system that reads real-time data from the field and processes it in the cloud, as well as a mobile application to monitor and operate the irrigation system remotely.

2.2.4 Robotics

Robotics in agriculture involves the use of automated machines to perform tasks such as harvesting, planting, and spraying. These robots are capable

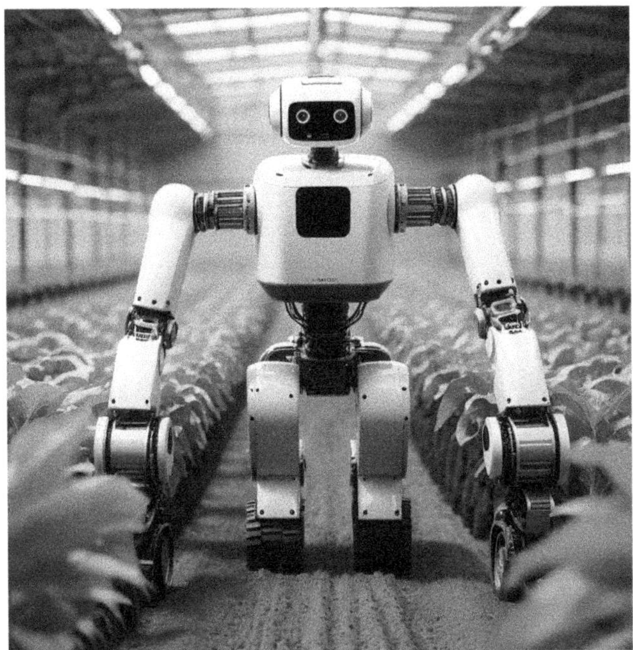

Figure 2.4 Application of robotics in agriculture automation.

of continuous operation with remarkable precision, diminishing the necessity for manual labor and enhancing productivity [24–26]. For example, autonomous tractors and harvesters can work tirelessly in the fields, ensuring timely and efficient completion of agricultural tasks as shown in Figure 2.4.

2.3 THE PROPOSED FRAMEWORK FOR AGRICULTURE AUTOMATION

The functionality of the intended framework is structured into four layers: installation of monitoring devices, deployment, data transmission, and processing. This system aims to enhance crop production by monitoring air quality, monitoring of the moisture of the soil, temperature, weather conditions, and pest control without human intervention. Additionally, the framework includes animal husbandry surveillance to monitor the health and count of animals. The main goal of the intended framework is to create an intelligent system aimed at enhancing agricultural productivity.

Figure 2.5 illustrates the process flowchart of the smart agriculture framework assisted by IoT and AI. The first operational layer is responsible for the installation of the monitoring devices. Sensors are employed

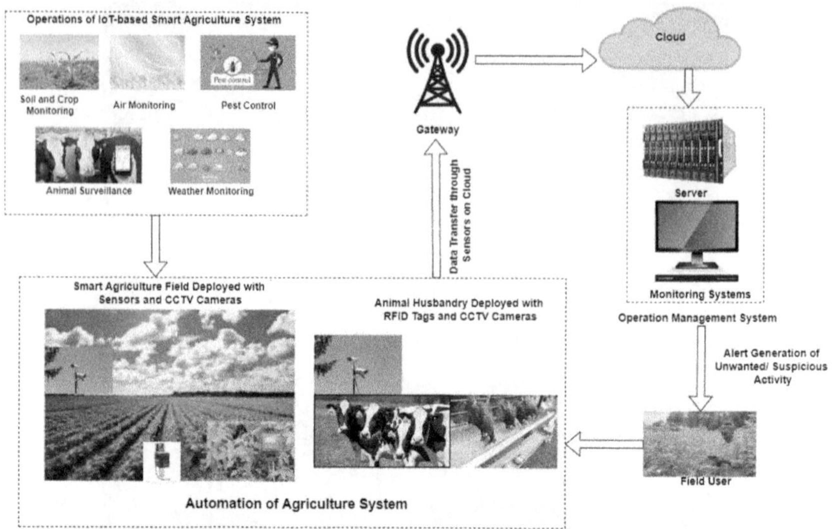

Figure 2.5 The proposed AI and IoT assisted framework for agricultural automation.

to measure air humidity, soil moisture, wind direction, and wind speed, gathering real-time data from agricultural fields. CCTV cameras are strategically placed in fields and livestock areas to monitor for any unauthorized or skeptical activities. Furthermore, RFID tags are utilized alongside CCTV cameras to track and monitor animals, facilitating the location of missing livestock. Images captured from the field assist in identifying potential pest infestations.

The second layer is the implementation layer, responsible for executing agricultural automation techniques. Computer vision and image processing techniques are utilized for animal surveillance and pest control. Sensors estimate soil moisture levels, generating an alert if the moisture falls below a threshold, prompting the automatic activation of irrigation systems. Once the desired moisture level is reached, the system turns off. Likewise, air and weather monitoring are conducted using MQ135 and DHT11 sensors, with alerts sent to field users' mobile phones. The greenhouse flap automatically opens to maintain the required humidity and temperature based on sensor data. Surveillance monitors suspicious activities in fields and livestock areas, reducing the need for human intervention. Computer vision techniques detect pests in field images, triggering automatic pesticide spraying.

The third layer includes the data transmission and cloud analysis segment. It utilizes Arduino UNO-based microcontrollers and Raspberry

Pi to transmit sensor data to the cloud for analysis. Data is transmitted wirelessly from the collection point to the base station through a gateway. Using Internet Protocol (IP), the gathered data is then sent to the cloud for analysis and decision-making.

The final operational layer creates channels for specific field parameters, enabling frequent data monitoring and archiving with time and date stamps. The gateway node dispatches the recorded data to its designated channels. Through a web service, data can be monitored remotely from any location at any given time. Consistent monitoring of agricultural and animal husbandry activities guarantees prompt alert notifications when required.

2.3.1 Comparative analysis of the proposed framework with existing systems

Table 2.2 discusses the comparison between the proposed approach and other contemporary techniques. The proposed framework expands its range of functionalities to include cloud analysis, future-oriented data storage, smart devices, and more, aimed at automating agricultural operations.

Table 2.2 Comparative analysis of the proposed framework with existing systems

Author and Year	System Capabilities	Technology Used	Intelligent Devices	Cloud Infrastructure Assessment	Advanced Storage Solutions
Liqiang et al. [36], 2011	Monitoring of Crop	WSN	Y	N	N
Heble et al. [37], 2018	Monitoring of soil moisture, temperature, wind speed	IoT	Y	N	N
Haseeb et al [38], 2020	Monitoring of soil moisture, temperature, weather	WSN, IoT, Data Encryption	Y	Y	Y
Yang et al. [39], 2021	Monitoring of crop & soil, weather, air	Sensor Networks, IoT	Y	Y	Y
Mini et al. [40], 2023	Monitoring of soil	WSN, IoT	Y	N	N
Proposed Framework, 2024	Monitoring of crop & soil, weather, air, animal surveillance, pest control	Computer Vision, IoT, Sensor Networks, Image Processing,	Y	Y	Y

Note: *Y=Yes, N=No, WSN: Wireless Sensor Networks.

2.4 IMPORTANCE OF AGRICULTURE AUTOMATION

The need for smart and sustainable agriculture arises from the growing global population and the consequent increase in food demand. As per the United Nations, projections indicate that the global population will exceed nine billion by the year 2050 [41]. In order to fulfill the nutritional needs of this expanding population, agricultural practices must become more efficient, sustainable, and resilient.

2.4.1 Enhancing productivity

Smart agriculture systems leverage advanced technologies to optimize every aspect of farming, from soil preparation to harvesting. By collecting and analyzing data in real-time, these systems enable precise control over farming operations, leading to higher productivity and better crop quality.

2.4.2 Reducing environmental impact

Sustainable agriculture aims to minimize the environmental footprint of farming activities. Automation technologies help achieve this by reducing the use of water, fertilizers, and pesticides through precise application. As an example, intelligent irrigation systems can guarantee crops receive optimal water quantities at precise timings, diminishing water wastage and fostering sustainable water management practices.

2.4.3 Addressing labor shortages

The agricultural sector often faces labor shortages, particularly during peak seasons. Automation can alleviate this problem by performing labor-intensive tasks such as planting, weeding, and harvesting. This not only ensures timely completion of these tasks but also reduces the reliance on manual labor.

2.5 ISSUES IN AGRICULTURE AUTOMATION

Agriculture automation holds the promise of enhancing productivity, efficiency, and sustainability in farming practices. Nonetheless, it also poses numerous challenges that require attention and resolution. These challenges can be classified into three main categories: technical challenges, business issues, and human factors. Below is a detailed examination of these issues.

2.5.1 Technical issues

Implementation Challenges: Implementing automated systems in agriculture requires a variety of sophisticated resources. This includes high-quality sensors, cameras for image capture, powerful processors, and substantial memory for fast execution in computer vision-based systems. IoT-based applications also require high-speed internet, reliable semiconductor devices, and extensive cloud storage capabilities. These requirements pose significant barriers to the successful deployment of agricultural automation.

System Reliability: The dependability of automated systems is critical, as any failure can lead to substantial disruptions in agricultural operations. Automated equipment is often used in harsh outdoor environments, which can cause degradation of sensors, lenses, and other components. Ensuring the physical durability and reliability of these systems in variable and challenging environmental conditions is a major technical hurdle.

Data Management: Effective automation relies heavily on data collection and management. AI-based systems, in particular, require large datasets for training and operation. Collecting, storing, and processing this data can be challenging, especially given the inconsistent adoption of automation technologies among farmers. Additionally, ensuring data accuracy, security, and privacy adds to the complexity of data management in agriculture automation.

Interoperability: Integrating various automated systems and ensuring they work seamlessly together is another significant technical challenge. Different devices and platforms need to communicate and share data effectively. Achieving interoperability requires standardized protocols and compatibility across diverse systems, which can be difficult to implement and maintain.

2.5.2 Business issues

High Costs: The initial investment required for automation in agriculture is substantial. Costs include purchasing hardware, setting up infrastructure, ongoing maintenance, data management services, and training personnel. The elevated expenses may pose a hurdle, especially for small-scale farmers, making it difficult to justify the investment against the anticipated returns.

Return on Investment (ROI): Calculating the ROI for automated systems in agriculture can be complex. The benefits, such as increased efficiency, yield, and cost savings, may take time to materialize. Farmers and agribusinesses need clear, demonstrable evidence of the financial advantages of adopting automation technologies, which can be challenging to provide due to variability in agricultural conditions and practices.

Market Dynamics: The agricultural technology market is highly competitive and rapidly evolving. Companies developing automation solutions must keep pace with technological advancements and changing market demands. This requires continuous innovation and significant investment in research and development, which can be risky and expensive.

2.5.3 Human factors

Resistance to Change: Farmers who have practiced traditional methods for generations may hesitate to embrace new automated technologies. This reluctance can arise from distrust in unfamiliar systems, fear of the unknown, and concerns about how these technologies might challenge their expertise and traditional knowledge.

Skill Gap: The successful deployment and operation of automated systems require new skills and knowledge. Farmers and agricultural laborers require training to proficiently utilize and sustain these technologies. Bridging this skill gap involves substantial educational efforts and ongoing support, which can be resource intensive.

Accessibility and Equity: Ensuring that all farmers, especially those in remote and rural areas, have access to automation technologies is a significant challenge. Infrastructure limitations, such as lack of internet connectivity and electricity, can hinder the adoption of these technologies. Additionally, there is a need to ensure that small-scale and resource-poor farmers can benefit from automation, avoiding a digital divide that exacerbates existing inequalities.

Cultural and Social Factors: The adoption of automation technologies must also consider cultural and social factors. Farmers' practices are often deeply rooted in their cultural and social contexts. Efforts to promote automation must be sensitive to these contexts and seek to integrate new technologies in ways that respect and enhance traditional practices rather than displacing them.

Agriculture automation offers significant potential benefits, it also presents substantial technical, business, and human challenges. Addressing these issues will require coordinated efforts from technology developers, educators, policymakers, and the agricultural community to guarantee that the advantages of automation are realized and accessible to all farmers.

2.6 CONCLUSION AND FUTURE OUTLOOK

The projected global population of ten billion by 2050, as forecasted by the United Nations, underscores the urgent need for advancements in agriculture. With an additional two billion people to feed, there will be heightened demand for high-quality, cost-effective agricultural products. This challenge is compounded by shrinking arable land due to urbanization. Innovative approaches are essential to meet these evolving demands. Computer vision and image processing algorithms play a pivotal role in advancing smart agriculture. These technologies aid in insect control, weed eradication, optimizing yield production, and identifying plant species. Coupled with Internet of Things (IoT), Robotics, and Cloud Computing, they offer transformative potential. Precision farming, Smart Irrigation, Smart Greenhouse management, and Livestock Monitoring exemplify how these technologies enhance productivity and efficiency. Integration of IoT, Cloud Computing, Big Data Analytics, Robotics, Computer Vision, and Artificial Intelligence presents vast opportunities. These technologies provide solutions for resource management, pest control, and crop optimization, promoting sustainable agricultural practices.

Cutting-edge tools such as UAVs, sensors, drones, RFID tags, and smartphones enable real-time monitoring and data-driven decision-making. They empower farmers to optimize operations and make informed choices. The future of agriculture hinges on embracing technological advancements to sustainably feed a growing global population. Continued investment in research and development is crucial to fully leverage technology in shaping agriculture's future.

REFERENCES

[1] L. Taiz, "Agriculture, plant physiology, and human population growth: Past, present, and future," *Theoretical and Experimental Plant Physiology*, 25, 167–181, 2013.

[2] Y. Edan, G. Adamides, & R. Oberti, *"Agriculture Automation,"* Springer Handbook of Automation, 1055–1078, 2023.

[3] C. Brewster, I. Roussaki, N. Kalatzis, K. Doolin, & K. Ellis, "IoT in agriculture: Designing a Europe-wide large-scale pilot," *IEEE Communications Magazine*, 55(9), 26–33, 2017.

[4] S. Anwarul, T. Misra, & D. Srivastava, "An IoT & AI-assisted framework for agriculture automation," In *2022 10th International Conference on Reliability, Infocom Technologies and Optimization (Trends and Future Directions)(ICRITO)* (pp. 1–6). IEEE, 2022.

[5] S. Anwarul, & D. Joshi, "Deep learning with tensorflow," In Mehul Mahrishi & Kamal Kant Hiran (eds.), *Machine Learning and Deep Learning in Real-Time Applications*, IGI Global, pp. 96–120, 2020.

[6] S. Anwarul, "An efficient minimum spanning tree-based color image segmentation approach," In *International Advanced Computing Conference* (pp. 588–598), Springer International Publishing, 2021.

[7] K. Jha, A. Doshi, P. Patel, & M. Shah, "A comprehensive review on automation in agriculture using artificial intelligence," *Artificial Intelligence in Agriculture*, 2, 1–12, 2019.

[8] W. S. Kim, W. S. Lee, & Y. J. Kim, "A review of the applications of the internet of things (IoT) for agricultural automation," *Journal of Biosystems Engineering*, 45, 385–400, 2020.

[9] M. H. Saleem, J. Potgieter, & K. M. Arif, "Automation in agriculture by machine and deep learning techniques: A review of recent developments, " *Precision Agriculture*, 22(6), 2053–2091, 2021.

[10] K. Phasinam, T. Kassanuk, P. P. Shinde, C. M. Thakar, D. K. Sharma, M. K. Mohiddin, & A. W. Rahmani, "Application of IoT and cloud computing in automation of agriculture irrigation, " *Journal of Food Quality*, 1–8, 2022.

[11] H. Tian, T. Wang, Y. Liu, X. Qiao, & Y. Li, "Computer vision technology in agricultural automation—A review, " *Information Processing in Agriculture*, 7(1), 1–19, 2020.

[12] Y. Jararweh, S. Fatima, M. Jarrah, & S. AlZu'bi, "Smart and sustainable agriculture: Fundamentals, enabling technologies, and future directions," *Computers and Electrical Engineering*, 110, 108799, 2023.

[13] E. Alreshidi, "Smart sustainable agriculture (SSA) solution underpinned by internet of things (IoT) and artificial intelligence (AI)," arXiv preprint arXiv:1906.03106, 2019.

[14] D. Soni, D. Srivastava, A. Bhatt, A. Aggarwal, S. Kumar, & M. A. Shah, "An empirical client cloud environment to secure data communication with alert protocol," *Mathematical Problems in Engineering*, 2022, 4696649, 2022.

[15] A. Aggarwal, S. Kumar, A. Bhatt, & M. A. Shah, "Solving user priority in cloud computing using enhanced optimization algorithm in workflow scheduling," *Computational Intelligence and Neuroscience*, 2022, 7855532, 2022.

[16] A. Rehman, T. Saba, M. Kashif, S. M. Fati, S. A. Bahaj, & H. Chaudhry, "A revisit of internet of things technologies for monitoring and control strategies in smart agriculture," *Agronomy*, 12(1), 127, 2022.

[17] E. Biffis, & E. Chavez, "Satellite data and machine learning for weather risk management and food security," *Risk Analysis*, 37(8), 1508–1521, 2017.

[18] S. Anwarul, & S. Agarwal, "Image enciphering using modified AES with secure key transmission," In *Proc. of the Int. Conf. on Communication and Computing Systems (ICCCS)* (p. 137), 2017. CRC Press.

[19] M. Bagheri, K. Al-Jabery, D. Wunsch, & J. G. Burken, "Examining plant uptake and translocation of emerging contaminants using machine learning: Implications to food security," *Science of the Total Environment*, 698, 133999, 2020.

[20] S. Anwarul, M. Mohan, & R. Agarwal, "An unprecedented approach for deep learning assisted web application to diagnose plant disease," *Procedia Computer Science*, 218, 1444–1453, 2023.

[21] L. Zhu, P. Spachos, E. Pensini, & K. N. Plataniotis, "Deep learning and machine vision for food processing: A survey," *Current Research in Food Science*, 4, 233–249, 2021.

[22] S. K. Choudhary, R. S. Jadoun, & H. L. Mandoriya, "Role of cloud computing technology in agriculture fields," *Computing*, 7(3), 1–7, 2016.

[23] C. Cambra, S. Sendra, J. Lloret, & L. Garcia, "An IoT service-oriented system for agriculture monitoring," In *2017 IEEE International Conference on Communications (ICC)* (pp. 1–6). IEEE, 2017.

[24] T. M. Shah, D. P. B Nasika, & R. Otterpohl, "Plant and weed identifier robot as an agroecological tool using artificial neural networks for image identification," *Agriculture*, 11(3), 222, 2021.

[25] M. Thanjaivadivel, "Agribot-plant disease predictor," *Turkish Journal of Computer and Mathematics Education (TURCOMAT)*, 12(9), 254–264, 2021.

[26] S. Sowmiya, "Robotics in Agriculture: Transforming Farming for a Sustainable Future," 2023. Accessed on 17-May 2024 from www.linkedin.com/pulse/robotics-agriculture-transforming-farming-sustainable-sowmiya-s/

[27] M. Kumar, S. Gupta, X. Z. Gao, & A. Singh, "Plant species recognition using morphological features and adaptive boosting methodology," *IEEE Access*, 7, 163912–163918, 2019.

[28] P. S. Mahore, & A. A. Bardekar, "Crop yield prediction using different machine learning techniques," *International Journal of Scientific Research in Computer Science, Engineering and Information Technology*, 7, 561–569, 2021.

[29] S. J. Dorman, M. W. Kudenov, A. J. Lytle, E. H. Griffith, & A. S. Huseth, "Computer vision for detecting field-evolved lepidopteran resistance to Bt maize," *Pest Management Science*, 77(11), 5236–5245, 2021.

[30] M. Roopaei, P. Rad, & K. K. R. Choo, "Cloud of things in smart agriculture: Intelligent irrigation monitoring by thermal imaging," *IEEE Cloud Computing*, 4(1), 10–15, 2017.

[31] S. Namani, & B. Gonen, "Smart agriculture based on IoT and cloud computing," In *2020 3rd International Conference on Information and Computer Technologies (ICICT)* (pp. 553–556). IEEE, 2020.

[32] D. Raghuvanshi, A. Roy, & V. Panwar, "IoT Based Smart Agriculture System," *International Journal of Research in Engineering and Science (IJRES)*, 9(6), 2021.

[33] Y. Ge, Y. Xiong, G. L. Tenorio, & P. J. From, "Fruit localization and environment perception for strawberry harvesting robots," *IEEE Access*, 7, 147642–147652, 2019.

[34] M. Hussain, S. H. A. Naqvi, S. H. Khan, & M. Farhan, "An Intelligent Autonomous Robotic System for Precision Farming," In *2020 3rd International Conference on Intelligent Autonomous Systems (ICoIAS)* (pp. 133–139). IEEE, 2020.

[35] P. Kumar, & G. Ashok, "Design and fabrication of smart seed sowing robot," *Materials Today: Proceedings*, 39, 354–358, 2021.

[36] Z. Liqiang, Y. Shouyi, L. Leibo, Z. Zhen, & W. Shaojun, A crop monitoring system based on wireless sensor network," *Procedia Environmental Sciences*, 11, 558–565, 2011.

[37] S. Heble, A. Kumar, K. V. D. Prasad, S. Samirana, P. Rajalakshmi, & U. B. Desai, "A low power IoT network for smart agriculture," *In 2018 IEEE 4th World Forum on Internet of Things (WF-IoT)* (pp. 609–614). IEEE, 2018.

[38] K. Haseeb, I. Ud Din, A. Almogren, & N. Islam, "An energy efficient and secure IoT-based WSN framework: An application to smart agriculture," *Sensors*, 20(7), 2081, 2020.

[39] J. Yang, A. Sharma, & R. Kumar, "IoT-based framework for smart agriculture," *International Journal of Agricultural and Environmental Information Systems (IJAEIS)*, 12(2), 1–14, 2021.

[40] A. D. Mini, M. A. S. Anuradha, G. S. R. Asha, J. S. S Rekha, S. Kamble, & M. Kulkarni, "IoT based smart agriculture monitoring system," *International Research Journal of Engineering and Technology*, 10(4), 1442–1448, 2023.

[41] S. Sarfraz, F. Ali, A. Hameed, Z. Ahmad, & K. Riaz, "Sustainable agriculture through technological innovations," In *Sustainable agriculture in the era of the OMICs revolution* (pp. 223–239). Springer International Publishing, 2023.

Chapter 3

Enhancing face recognition accuracy in authentication systems through hyperparameter tuning of deep learning models

Shahina Anwarul

3.1 INTRODUCTION

Biometric systems aim to authenticate individuals by utilizing one or multiple distinctive biometric characteristics, such as facial features, iris patterns, fingerprints, and other similar traits. The biometric traits can be classified into behavioral and physiological traits, as shown in Figure 3.1. Traditional authentication methods, such as identification cards and passwords, are often lost or stolen, while biometric-based systems improve security over traditional methods. Broadly, biometric applications can be categorized into three primary categories: verification, identification, and screening. Verification involves comparing an individual's biometric data with the stored data to validate their identity (referred to as one-to-one matching). The second category entails comparing an individual's biometric traits with the traits of various individuals stored in the system (known as one-to-many matching). In the last category, a small number of target persons are matched with unknown persons from a large group of people (i.e., many-to-some matching).

There is a growing need for biometric security solutions to protect against fraud, theft, and other risks. Face Recognition (FR) holds a crucial position in biometrics-based security techniques and has proven to be a valuable tool across a diverse range of applications, including disease identification, forensic analysis, secure transactions, missing person searches, e-passport identification, mask recognition, and more [1–3]. Face Recognition has drawn the most attention from researchers among the many biometric applications in recent years since it is more covert, non-intrusive, and requires less human involvement than other biometrics like the iris, fingerprint, or palmprint. The FR process involves analyzing and comparing essential facial features and expressions, aiming to enhance the intelligence and safety of our world. This technology finds applications in authentication and surveillance, allowing for the identification of individuals and, when needed, the detection of suspects or suspicious behavior. Face Recognition is a crucial component for person identification. The automated FR system

DOI: 10.1201/9781003518075-3

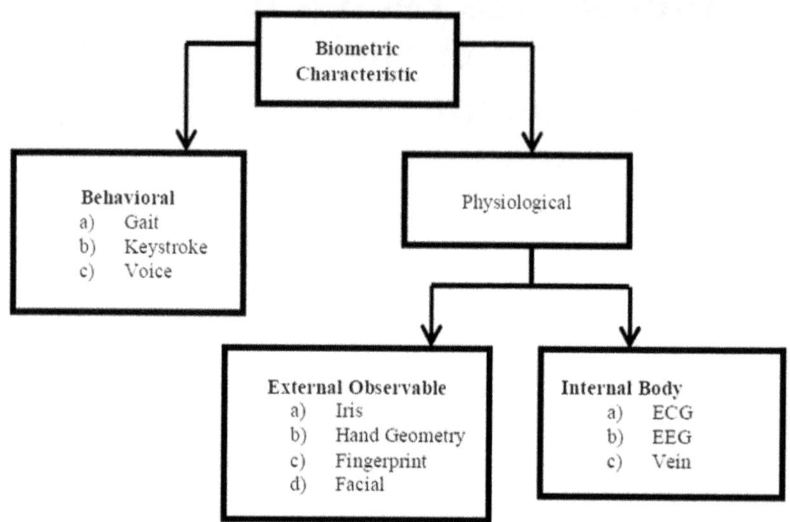

Figure 3.1 Classification of biometric characteristics.

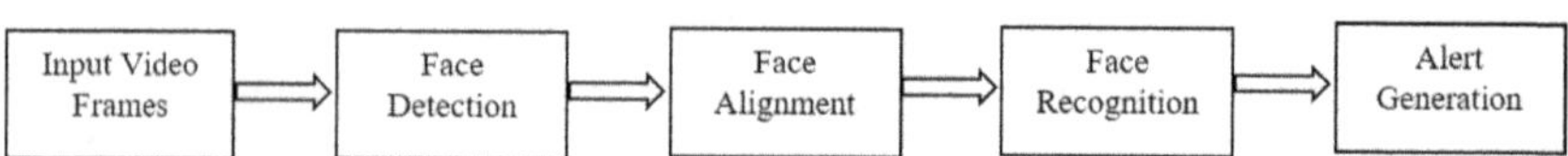

Figure 3.2 The block diagram of an automated authentication FR system.

encompasses fundamental steps such as face detection, face alignment, face recognition, and alert generation, as depicted in Figure 3.2. An automated Face Recognition (FR) system integrates several pivotal steps to facilitate its operation effectively. Initially, the system performs face detection, which involves identifying and localizing human faces within images or video frames using advanced algorithms like Haar cascades or Convolutional Neural Networks (CNNs). Following detection, the system proceeds to face alignment, a crucial process that normalizes the orientation and positioning of detected faces to a standardized format. This alignment minimizes variations caused by factors such as pose, scale, or rotation, thereby enhancing the accuracy of subsequent tasks. Subsequently, face recognition takes place, where the system compares the extracted facial features of the aligned face with stored data in a database to identify individuals. Techniques such as Principal Component Analysis (PCA) or deep learning models such as FaceNet are commonly employed for accurate recognition. Upon successful identification, the system may trigger alert generation based on predefined rules. Alerts could signify the presence of recognized individuals, potential security threats, or facilitate personalized interactions in applications ranging from access control systems to surveillance and customer service environments. Together, these integrated steps form the foundational framework of automated FR systems, enabling efficient and reliable deployment across diverse operational scenarios.

3.2 LITERATURE REVIEW

The task of FR in photos and videos is certainly difficult, and reaching 100% accuracy is a constant endeavor due to different factors influencing FR system performance. Despite intensive efforts, sufficient results have yet to be obtained, owing mostly to the numerous factors influencing the accuracy of these systems. Numerous studies have found that occlusion, low resolution, noise, illumination, position change, face expression, aging, and plastic surgery have an impact on recognition accuracy [4–6]. These components are categorized into two parts: internal and extrinsic factors [4]. Intrinsic factors are the physical qualities of the human face that affect recognition accuracy, such as aging, facial expression, and plastic surgery. Extrinsic factors, on the other hand, alter the facial appearance and include occlusion, low resolution, noise, lighting, and position change, as shown in Figure 3.3.

Extensive research has been done in the area of face detection and recognition. Traditional approaches for face recognition primarily involve

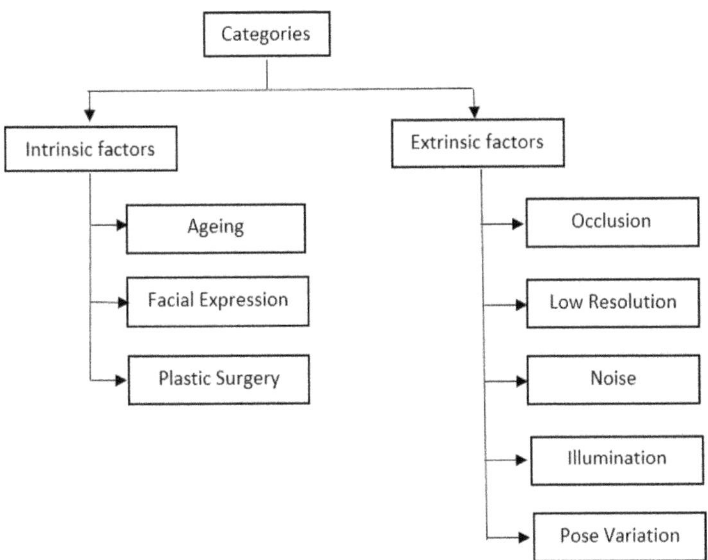

Figure 3.3 The classification of the factors affecting FR accuracy.

the use of Principal Component Analysis (PCA), achieving accuracy rates ranging from 69% to 95% in controlled environments [7]. PCA has also been combined with other methods such as Singular Value Decomposition (SVD) and Fisherface techniques, resulting in recognition rates of 93.92% and 99.5% for frontal faces [8]. Furthermore, researchers also investigated non-frontal FR techniques, such as mirroring, stretching, segmentation, and Three-Dimensional (3D) operations [9, 10]. However, the effectiveness of these methods tends to decline when facial images are captured in challenging environmental conditions, such as inadequate lighting, low-resolution cameras, and occluded facial images [11–13]. With the emergence of deep learning [14, 15], the constraints of traditional methods have been surpassed [16]. However, deep learning techniques still face significant challenges such as their reliance on vast amounts of data and high-performance computing systems, often accelerated by Graphical Processing Units (GPUs) [17, 18]. Acquiring large, annotated facial datasets for face recognition tasks remains difficult due to privacy concerns [19]. A proposed solution to these challenges is deep ensemble transfer learning [20], which offers efficiencies in both time and resource utilization. Transfer learning leverages pretrained model features, avoiding the laborious process of building and training a model from scratch [21]. Instead, it utilizes pretrained model weights to adapt and train new models for specific tasks. Ensemble learning is employed to enhance recognition accuracy by averaging the weights of multiple deep-learning models. It combines the benefits of deep learning and ensemble learning to achieve improved generalization performance in the final model [22].

3.2.1 Motivation

Face detection and recognition play a crucial role in authentication systems based on biometric data, serving purposes in both authentication processes and surveillance. As scams and fraudulent activities continue to rise, facial recognition has become an essential system for ensuring security. Extensive research has been conducted globally to advance this field; however, despite continuous efforts, there is still a lack of robust and effective automated systems capable of performing well in both controlled and uncontrolled environments. Face Recognition has always been a highly intricate and demanding task, as it strives to replicate the human ability to perceive and identify faces. Nonetheless, human capabilities have limitations when dealing with various ambiguous phenomena. Hence, there is a need for an automated electronic system with high recognition accuracy and fast processing capabilities. The demand for biometric security systems has witnessed a substantial surge in recent times, driven by the need for enhanced protection and security against fraud, theft, and other related threats. Among the various biometric-based systems, Face Recognition has emerged as a prominent and effective solution. It serves various applications, including forensics, criminal identification, surveillance, and fraud prevention, as it can authenticate an individual's identity and recognize individuals in different scenarios. Face Recognition system is used in banks, railway stations, airports, and other public places as a security control system where Closed-Circuit Television (CCTV) cameras are leased to identify individuals. It is also used in other sectors such as education, healthcare, media and entertainment, *etc.*, as illustrated in Figure 3.4 [23]. Video surveillance recordings can assist in identifying suspects at crime scenes. Continuously monitoring surveillance videos demands sustained visual attention and can be monotonous, increasing the likelihood of errors. Implementing automated surveillance systems equipped with intelligent algorithms to monitor activities and trigger alarms when needed can establish a highly effective security solution. In these real-time scenarios, there is a high possibility that the captured image has a large pose variation, faces are obscured by glasses, clothes, *etc.*, the lighting effect of the image might be dark, the facial expression might be different, *etc.* These are the factors that contribute to the deterioration in facial recognition accuracy. Therefore, an effective automated facial recognition system that offers high accuracy with minimal computational cost is the need of the hour.

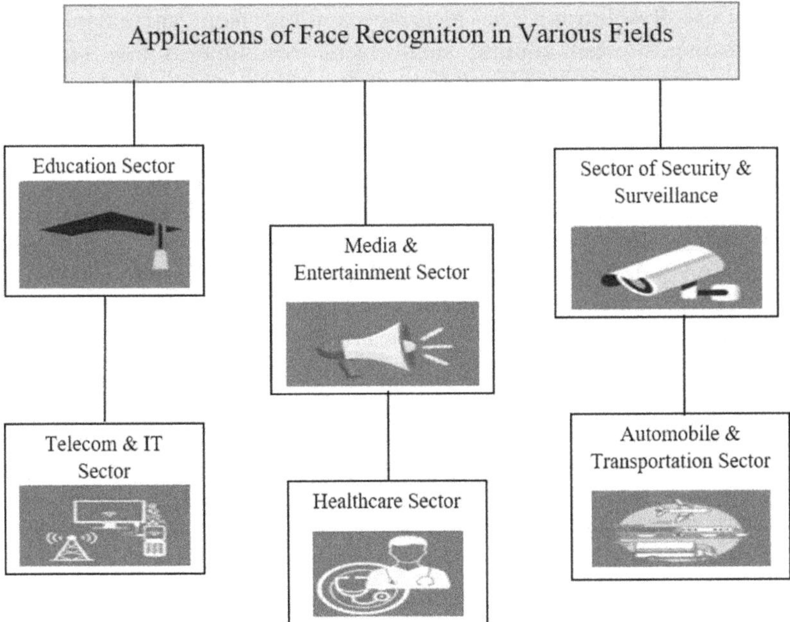

Figure 3.4 Applications of FR in various sectors.

3.2.2 Challenging areas of face recognition

Face recognition from images and videos presents significant challenges, and extensive research has been conducted to achieve high precision. However, satisfactory results are yet to be attained due to various factors that affect the performance of these systems. These factors include occlusion, low resolution, noise, illumination, pose variation, expressions, aging, and plastic surgery [4, 24]. These can be classified into two main groups: intrinsic and extrinsic factors [4]. Intrinsic factors are tied to the inherent attributes of the human face, including aging, facial expressions, and plastic surgery, directly influencing the system. Conversely, extrinsic factors entail alterations in facial appearance like occlusion, low resolution, noise, illumination, and pose variation.

a) **Occlusion:** Partial occlusion emerges as a notable obstacle in the realm of face recognition endeavors. The concealment of specific facial features impedes the precise identification of individuals. For instance, eyeglasses or sunglasses can obscure the eyes; earrings or hair might veil the ears; scarves could shroud a substantial portion of the face; and facial hair like moustaches and beards might obscure significant facial attributes. These factors have a detrimental effect on the performance of face recognition systems. Researchers have been investigating various approaches to address these challenges [25, 26].

b) **Low Resolution:** The pictures captured from surveillance video cameras often contain small faces, resulting in low resolution. Comparing a low-resolution query image with a high-resolution gallery image poses a significant challenge. The limited data in a low-resolution image leads to the loss of many important details, which can significantly degrade recognition accuracy. Researchers have been exploring various approaches to address this issue [25, 27].

c) **Noise:** Digital images are susceptible to different types of noise, which can result in poor accuracy in detection and recognition tasks. The introduction of noise into images can occur through various means, depending on how the image is created. Pre-processing plays a crucial role in the overall face detection and recognition system [28].

d) **Illumination:** The changes in illumination significantly affect the performance of face recognition systems. Factors like background light, shadows, brightness, and contrast variations contribute to these fluctuations. Several approaches to addressing illumination-related challenges are discussed in [29–31].

e) **Pose Variation:** Pose variation poses a significant challenge for face recognition systems. Matching a profile face with a frontal face in the gallery requires frontal face reconstruction [12]. This reconstruction is necessary because dataset images typically contain frontal views, and matching non-frontal profile faces can lead to inaccurate results. Researchers have proposed various approaches to convert non-frontal faces to frontal faces, which can improve recognition accuracy [9, 32]. The detrimental impact of pose variation on algorithm performance is extensively discussed in the proposed approaches [33–35].

f) **Expressions:** Facial expressions play a crucial role in expressing our emotions. They can alter the facial geometry, and even a slight variation can introduce ambiguity for face recognition systems. Muscle contractions that occur quickly lead to changes in facial features like the mouth, cheeks, and eyebrows, which are all part of facial expressions. Ongoing research focuses on incorporating facial expressions into face recognition methods [29, 36].

g) **Aging:** Aging is a natural factor that significantly impacts face recognition systems, often posing challenges for algorithms. The face comprises various components, including skin tissues, facial muscles, and bones. When muscles contract, they cause distortions in facial features. However, aging brings about substantial changes in facial appearance, such as changes in facial texture (*e.g.*, wrinkles) and face shape over time. Face recognition systems should be capable of addressing these changes [37, 38].

h) **Plastic Surgery:** Plastic surgery is another significant factor that can impact the accuracy of face recognition. Incidents have occurred where individuals have undergone plastic surgery due to accidents, resulting in their faces becoming unrecognizable to existing face recognition systems. This factor is particularly relevant in cases where criminals attempt to alter their identities through plastic surgery. Thus, as emphasized in [39], there is a requirement for an identification system that can recognize faces even after reconstructive surgery.

3.3 TECHNIQUES TO OPTIMIZE DEEP LEARNING MODELS

To enhance the efficiency of deep learning-based algorithms, the subsequent approaches can be implemented to mitigate the model's training time [40].

a) **Backpropagation:** Utilizing backpropagation techniques is an effective way to compute the gradient function during each iteration. This approach within deep learning employs gradient-based methods to address optimization challenges [41].

b) **Stochastic Gradient Descent (SGD):** It efficiently locates the optimal minimum through the utilization of convex functions by disregarding local minima. The determination of the optimal minimum across diverse trajectories is influenced by parameters such as step size, learning rate, and activation function values [42]. The mathematical equation for SGD to update the model's parameter is given in equation (3.1).

$$\theta_{i+1} = \theta_i - \eta \nabla J(\theta_i;\; x^{(i)}, y^{(i)}) \tag{3.1}$$

Here, θ_i represents the model's parameters at iteration i, η is the learning rate, and $\nabla J(\theta_i;\; x^{(i)}, y^{(i)})$ is the gradient of the loss function J.

c) **Learning Rate Decay:** Modifying the learning rate leads to a reduction in the training time of gradient descent algorithms while concurrently enhancing the model's overall performance. This approach finds extensive application due to its capacity to effect substantial changes during the initial training stages, subsequently gradually diminishing the learning rate. Moreover, this technique enables fine-tuning of weights in subsequent iterations and is mathematically represented by equation (3.2) [43].

$$k = i \times \frac{1}{1 + d \times \dfrac{k}{step\,size}} \tag{3.2}$$

Here, k is the learning rate, i is the initial learning rate at the beginning of training the mode, d is the decay rate at which the learning rate decreases, and step size is the number of epochs before each decay.

d) **Max-Pooling:** Across non-overlapping segments of the input layer, a pre-configured filter is employed to extract maximum values and generate the resulting output. The application of the max-pooling technique also brings about a reduction in computational expenses associated with learning multiple parameters [44, 45] and is mathematically represented as given in equation (3.3).

$$P = O_{max}^{n,n}(F) \tag{3.3}$$

Here, F is the input feature map of size $n \times n$ obtained from the previous convolutional layer.

e) **Dropout:** Tailored for the challenge of neural network overfitting, the dropout technique employs a strategy of randomly omitting units and their connections throughout the training phase. For a single neuron in a neural network layer, the output p after dropout is applied can be calculated using equation (3.4). This technique serves as an improved regularization approach, effectively curbing overfitting within neural networks and ameliorating generalization error [46]. In the realm of deep learning, this method garners superior results for supervised learning tasks [47].

$$\rho = \frac{1}{1-p} \cdot x \cdot d \tag{3.4}$$

Here, x is the output of the neuron before applying dropout, d is the binary dropout mask obtained from the Bernoulli distribution with probability p.

f) **Batch Normalization:** Batch normalization reduces covariate shift, which increases the learning rate of deep neural networks. During the training process, for each small batch, this method normalizes the input layer as the weights are adjusted. Enhanced network stability is achieved through the normalization of output from the final activation layer. Furthermore, batch normalization methodologies contribute to improved learning rates and a reduction in the required training epochs [48].

g) **Transfer Learning:** In this approach, a model initially trained for a particular task is adapted to undergo training for a comparable task. The knowledge acquired from addressing one challenge can be efficiently utilized to tackle another related issue. This process expedites advancements and enhances performance when addressing the second related task [21].

h) **Ensemble Learning:** In Machine Learning, ensemble techniques combine several models or classifiers to generate an ideal model that produces precise predictions for the intended result. Ensemble learning is employed to enhance recognition accuracy by averaging the weights of multiple deep learning models [49].

Based upon the aforementioned techniques for optimizing deep learning models, a comparison of their respective advantages and disadvantages is presented in Table 3.1.

3.4 PROPOSED METHODOLOGY

In proposed work, the impact of hyperparameter tuning such as learning rate, batch size, number of epochs, and data augmentation on face recognition accuracy is illustrated. Neurons serve as the computational units within a deep neural network (DNN), executing operations on data as it traverses the network. Each node within the DNN carries a weight value, learned during training, indicating its influence on prediction outcomes. These weights signify model parameters [50]. Hyperparameters, on the other hand, govern the training process. Crafting a Deep Neural Network (DNN) entails decisions like determining the hidden layer count between input and output layers and specifying node counts per layer. These aspects, while not directly

Table 3.1 Pros and cons of optimization techniques

S. No.	Technique	Description	Pros	Cons
1.	Back Propagation	Used in the optimization problems	Used to calculate the gradient	Susceptible to the effects of noisy data
2.	Stochastic Gradient Descent	Locate optimal minima in optimization problems	Prevents getting into local minima	Convergence time is large, demanding substantial computational resources
3.	Learning Rate Decay	Reduce the learning rate gradually	Enhancing the performance of the model helps reduce training time	Demanding significant computational resources
4.	Max-pooling	Downsampling technique for feature extraction	Reduces dimensionality and computational overhead	Considers only the maximum value of the region of an image, which may lead to an unacceptable result
5.	Dropout	Random deactivation of neurons during training	Prevents overfitting	Increases the training time required for the model to converge
6.	Batch Normalization	Nomalizing the activations of a layer within a mini-batch of data	Reduction in covariate shift, stable and faster convergence, and improved generalization	Increases implementation complexity and slows down the training of the model
7.	Transfer learning	Utilization of the knowledge of first model to resolve another problem	Handles data scarcity, improves performance of the model, and prevents overfitting	Limited flexibility (i.e., can work with similar types of problems)
8.	Ensemble learning	Prediction of each model is averaged to get the final prediction	Improves recognition accuracy	Computational overhead during training

tied to training data, are configuration variables. Hyperparameters typically remain fixed across tasks, while parameters change through training [50].

The endeavor to select optimal hyperparameter values for training a model using a tuned algorithm on a particular dataset is termed hyperparameter tuning. By optimizing model performance via a set of hyperparameters, the aim is to minimize a specified loss function, yielding improved results with fewer errors. Notably, the learning algorithm fine-tunes the loss based on input data, seeking the best solution within given constraints. Hyperparameters precisely shape this configuration. Inadequate adjustment of hyperparameters can lead to suboptimal outcomes even if model parameters are predicted accurately. In practice, the accuracy or confusion matrix might deteriorate [51].

For successful face recognition, meticulous hyperparameter tuning is crucial. The proposed model undergoes tuning via the judicious selection of pertinent parameters and hyperparameters for analysis and experimentation. This encompasses hyperparameters such as learning rate, batch size, epoch count, and data augmentation.

> **Learning rate:** The selection of an appropriate learning rate is of paramount importance. If the learning rate is overly large, it might lead to an overshoot of the optimal value; conversely, if it is excessively small, convergence to the optimal value may necessitate a protracted number of iterations. Thus, the Learning Rate Finder (LRF) curve [52] has been employed to ascertain the optimal learning rate for the model. The LRF curve is an invaluable tool for automatically identifying a suitable learning rate for any given model.
>
> **Batch size:** In the context of deep learning, a batch is a subset of the training dataset used to train the model in a single iteration. During training, instead of processing the entire dataset at once, the dataset is divided into smaller batches. Each batch is passed through the model, and the model's parameters (weights and biases) are updated based on the loss computed from that batch.
>
> **Epoch:** In deep learning, an epoch refers to a complete iteration through the entire training dataset. Within one epoch, the model evaluates each training example once, adjusting its internal parameters such as weights and biases based on the computed loss from its predictions. This iterative process is essential for the model to learn and refine its parameters, aiming to minimize errors and enhance overall performance.
>
> **Data augmentation:** Data augmentation, or data oversampling, serves as a strategy to amplify the dataset by generating virtual iterations of each image using a range of image transformation techniques. This practice is particularly valuable in the context of image classification tasks, as the augmentation process contributes to enhancing model performance by providing a broader and more varied dataset [53].

Algorithm 3.1 specifies the complete process of oversampling the dataset in this chapter. For every image, one augmentation technique (a_i) is randomly selected within configured thresholds, controlled by a parameter $'t'$, to apply a random magnitude of the transformation. If the dataset contains p samples in each class and the value of p varies within the classes of the dataset, then the proposed algorithm generates n target samples in each class to make it a class-balanced dataset. It selects the random augmentation a_i and applies all the r transformations to the randomly selected image. The output image I_{out} is generated after applying the transformations and added to the class C of the dataset. Through the implementation of oversampling techniques, the datasets are equalized, leading to a uniform distribution of images across all classes. The quantity of images for oversampling is determined by selecting the maximum image count among all classes within the dataset.

Algorithm 3.1: Algorithm for the process of data oversampling

---

Input: *Dataset D contains C different classes where each class consists of less than or equal to n unique samples, n is the maximum number of images in any class of the dataset, and A= [a1, a2, a3, a4, a5], where A is the set of all transformations applied on datasets.*

a1 = [centerCrop + ShiftScaleRotate + CLAHE]
a2 = [randomRotate90 + ShiftScaleRotate]
a3 = [flip + resize + randomBrightness]
a4 = [transpose]
a5 = [strongTransformation]

Output: *Dataset D contains C different classes where each class consists of n unique samples.*

1: **procedure** *Oversampling (D, n, A)*

2:     n ⟵ target number of images per class

3:     **for all** $C \in D$ **do**

4:         p ⟵ number of images in class C

5:         **while** $p \leq n$ **do**

6:             I ⟵ select one random image of C

7:             a_i ⟵ select one random transformation function from A

8:             r ⟵ transformations in a_i

9:             $I \longleftarrow I_{out}$

10:             **for all** $r \in a_i$ **do**

11:                 $I_{out} \longleftarrow r(I_{out})$

12:             **end for**

13:        $q \leftarrow I_{out}$

14:        $C \leftarrow C \cup q$

15:        $p \leftarrow p + 1$

16:        **end while**

17:   **end for**

18: **end procedure**

3.5 EXPERIMENTAL RESULTS AND DISCUSSION

The experiments utilized Teachable Machine, a user-friendly web tool created by Google, enabling model training in machine learning without requiring extensive coding expertise. By using their webcam, microphone, or by uploading images, users can create models to recognize objects, sounds, or poses, making machine learning accessible and easy to experiment with. The deep learning model is already available on the platform, and the results are obtained by adjusting hyperparameters such as epoch count, batch size, learning rate, and data augmentation for the model, as illustrated in Figures 3.5, 3.6, and 3.7. In Figure 3.5 (a), the trade-off between epoch count and accuracy is depicted when employing data augmentation. This figure illustrates how increasing the number of epochs affects the accuracy of the model when data augmentation techniques are applied during the training process. Common hyperparameter values were employed in the experiment: a batch size of 16, a learning rate set to 0.001, and a data split ratio of 450:80. Specifically, this ratio indicates that 450 images were allocated for training the model, while 80 images were reserved for testing its performance. Conversely, Figure 3.5 (b) showcases the results obtained without utilizing data augmentation. Common hyperparameter values were employed in the experiment: a batch size of 16, a learning rate set to 0.001, and a data split ratio of 192:37. Specifically, this ratio indicates that 192 images were allocated for training the model, while 37 images were reserved for testing its performance. This figure demonstrates the accuracy achieved with varying numbers of epochs when data augmentation techniques are not employed. Comparing both figures provides insights into the impact of data augmentation on the training process and the resultant accuracy of the model over different epochs. In Figure 3.6 (a), the trade-off between batch size and accuracy is depicted when employing data augmentation. This figure illustrates how increasing the batch size affects the accuracy of the model when data augmentation techniques are applied during the training process. Common hyperparameter values were employed in the experiment: an epoch count of 40, a learning rate set to

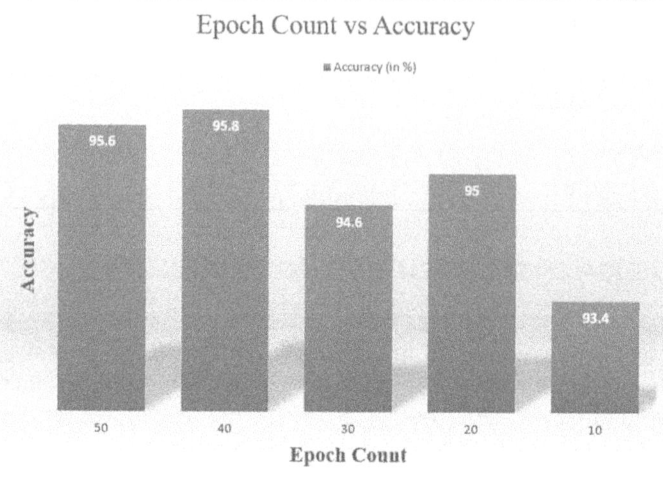

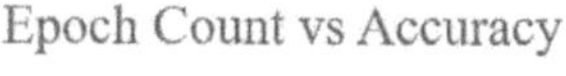

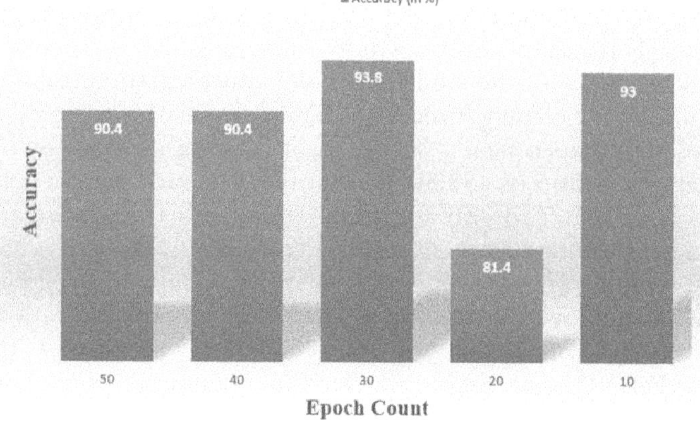

Figure 3.5 Experimental results after considering the variation in epoch count (a) With data augmentation (b) Without data augmentation.

0.001, and a data split ratio of 450:80. Specifically, this ratio indicates that 450 images were allocated for training the model, while 80 images were reserved for testing its performance. Conversely, Figure 3.6 (b) showcases the results obtained without utilizing data augmentation. Common hyperparameter values were employed in the experiment: an epoch count of 40, a learning rate set to 0.001, and a data split ratio of 192:37. Specifically, this ratio indicates that 192 images were allocated for training the model,

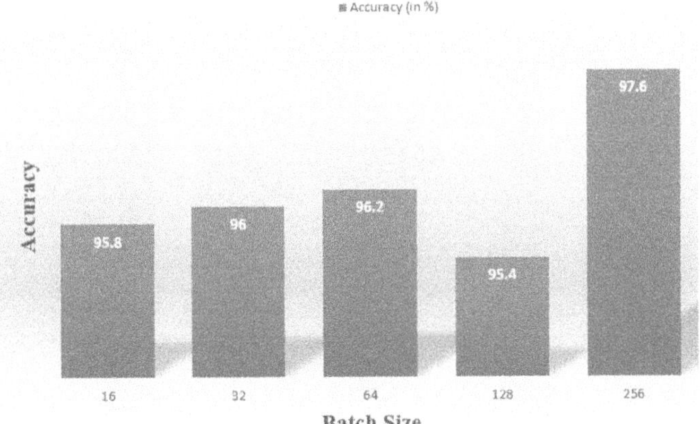

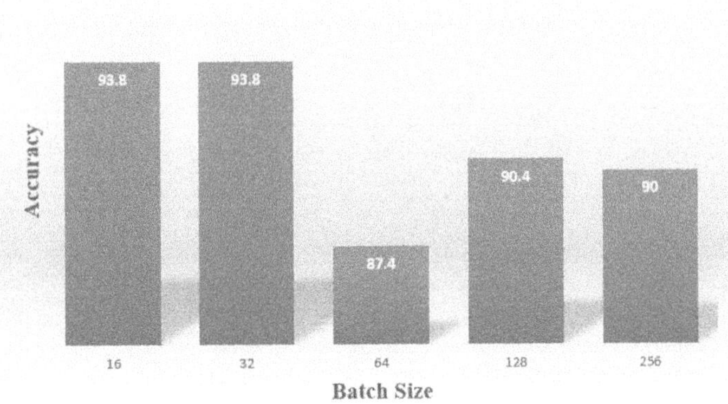

Figure 3.6 Experimental results after considering the variation in batch size (a) With data augmentation (b) Without data augmentation.

while 37 images were reserved for testing its performance. In Figure 3.7 (a), the trade-off between learning rate and accuracy is illustrated when employing data augmentation. This figure demonstrates how varying the learning rate impacts the accuracy of the model during the training process with the application of data augmentation techniques. The experiment utilized common hyperparameter values: a batch size of 256, a learning

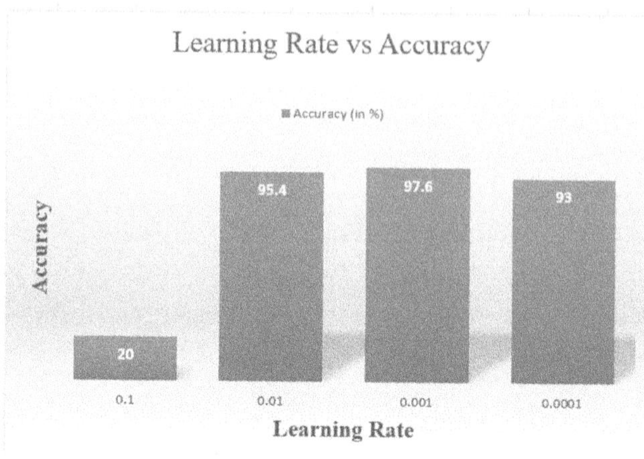

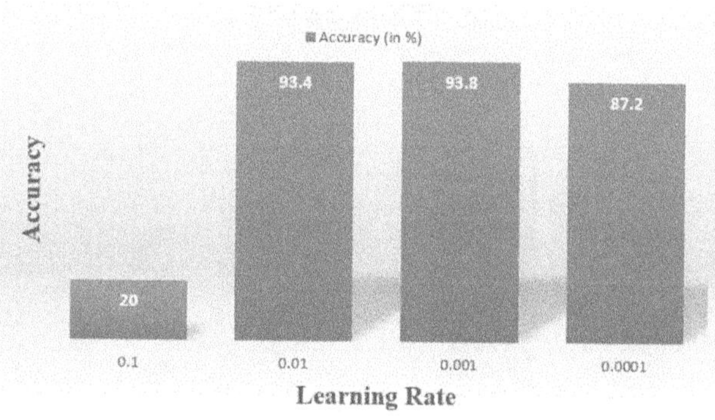

Figure 3.7 Experimental results after considering the variation in learning rate (a) With data augmentation (b) Without data augmentation.

rate set to 0.001, and a data split ratio of 450:80. Here, the ratio signifies that 450 images were used for training the model, while 80 images were set aside for testing its performance. Conversely, Figure 3.7 (b) presents results obtained without utilizing data augmentation. Similarly, the experiment employed common hyperparameter values: a batch size of 256, a learning rate set to 0.001, and a data split ratio of 192:37. In this case, 192 images were allocated for training, with 37 images reserved for testing the model's performance. These settings ensure consistency across the experiments and allow for meaningful comparisons of model performance under different training conditions.

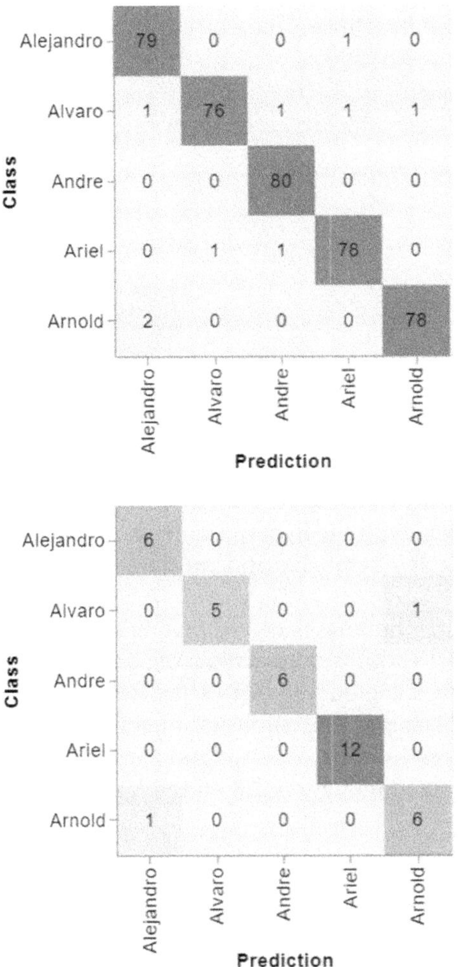

Figure 3.8 Confusion matrix (a) With data augmentation (b) Without data augmentation.

Sample images for the experiments were taken from the LFW dataset [54]. Five classes from the dataset were considered for experimental purposes. Experiments were conducted with and without data augmentation. A total of 229 images were used without data augmentation, while 2,650 images (530 images per class) were used after applying data augmentation. The dataset was split with approximately 84% of the images used for training and 16% for testing.

The highest accuracy of 97.6% was achieved with the hyperparameters: epoch count of 40, learning rate of 0.001, batch size of 256, and data

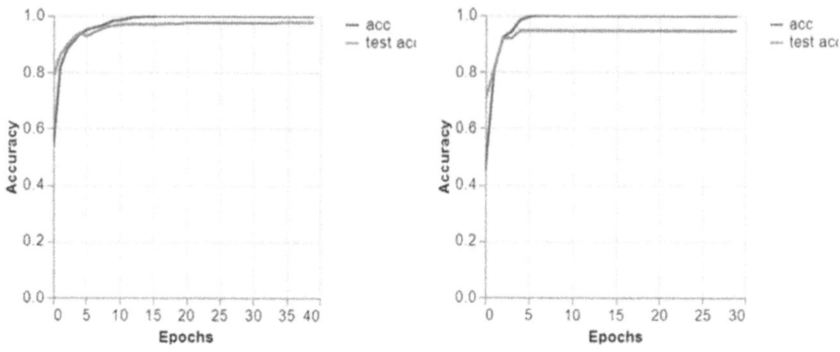

Figure 3.9 Graph between training and testing accuracy (a) With data augmentation (b) Without data augmentation.

augmentation, as shown in Figure 3.7 (a). Similarly, the highest accuracy of 93.8% was achieved with the hyperparameters: epoch count of 30, learning rate of 0.001, batch size of 32, and no data augmentation, as shown in Figure 3.7 (b).

The experimental findings suggest that employing data augmentation enhances the model's accuracy in recognizing patterns. A very small learning rate does not allow the model to learn effectively, and a very large learning rate also hinders learning. The confusion matrix and the graph showing the relationship between training and validation accuracy at the point of highest accuracy are presented in Figures 3.8 and 3.9, respectively.

3.6 CONCLUSION AND FUTURE SCOPE

In conclusion, this chapter has demonstrated the substantial impact of hyperparameter tuning on the accuracy of face recognition deep learning model. By meticulously adjusting key parameters, we have shown that it is possible to significantly enhance model performance, leading to more precise and reliable face recognition systems. This optimization process is essential for developing advanced models that meet the demands of real-world applications.

Looking ahead, the future scope of this research includes exploring automated hyperparameter optimization techniques, such as Bayesian optimization and genetic algorithms, to further streamline and improve the tuning process. Additionally, investigating the interplay between hyperparameter tuning and emerging deep learning architectures could yield even greater advancements in face recognition accuracy. Continuous innovation in this field will be crucial in addressing the evolving challenges in security, authentication, and other domains relying on robust face recognition technologies.

REFERENCES

[1] K. Xiao, Y. Tian, Y. Lu, Y. Lai, and X. Wang, "Quality assessment-based iris and face fusion recognition with dynamic weight," *The Visual Computer*, vol. 38, no. 5, pp. 1–13, 2022.

[2] N. Min-Allah, F. Jan, and S. Alrashed, "Pupil detection schemes in human eye: a review," *Multimedia Systems*, vol. 27, no. 4, pp. 753–777, 2021.

[3] R. S. Chowhan and R. Tanwar, "Password-less authentication: methods for user verification and identification to login securely over remote sites," in Muhammad Salman Khan (ed.), *Machine Learning and Cognitive Science Applications in Cyber Security*, IGI global, pp. 190–212, 2019.

[4] S. Anwarul and S. Dahiya, "A comprehensive review on face recognition methods and factors affecting facial recognition accuracy," in *Proceedings of ICRIC 2019: Recent Innovations in Computing*, Springer, pp. 495–514, 2019.

[5] S. Anwarul and S. Agarwal, "Image enciphering using modified AES with secure key transmission," in *Proc. of the Int. Conf. on Communication and Computing Systems (ICCCS)*, Taylor & Francis, p. 137, 2017.

[6] S. Anwarul, T. Choudhury, and S. Dahiya, "A novel hybrid ensemble convolutional neural network for face recognition by optimizing hyperparameters," *Nonlinear Engineering*, vol. 12, no. 1, pp. 20220290, 2023.

[7] A. Khan et al., "Forensic video analysis: Passive tracking system for automated Person of Interest (POI) localization," *IEEE Access*, vol. 6, pp. 43392–43403, 2018.

[8] J. Dhamija, T. Choudhury, P. Kumar, and Y. S. Rathore, "An advancement towards efficient face recognition using live video feed: 'For the future'," in *2017 3rd International Conference on Computational Intelligence and Networks (CINE)*, IEEE, pp. 53–56, 2017.

[9] J. Kavitha and T. T. Mirnalinee, "Automatic frontal face reconstruction approach for pose invariant face recognition," *Procedia Computer Science*, vol. 87, pp. 300–305, 2016.

[10] F. Liu, Q. Zhao, X. Liu, and D. Zeng, "Joint face alignment and 3D face reconstruction with application to face recognition," *IEEE Transactions on Pattern Analysis and Machine Intelligence*, vol. 42, no. 3, pp. 664–678, 2020.

[11] S. P. Mudunuri and S. Biswas, "Low resolution face recognition across variations in pose and illumination," *IEEE Transactions on Pattern Analysis and Machine Intelligence*, vol. 38, no. 5, pp. 1034–1040, 2016.

[12] Y. H. Huang and H. H. Chen, "Face recognition under low illumination via deep feature reconstruction network," in *2020 IEEE International Conference on Image Processing (ICIP)*, IEEE, pp. 2161–2165z, 2020.

[13] D. Zeng, R. Veldhuis, and L. Spreeuwers, "A survey of face recognition techniques under occlusion," *IET Biometrics*, vol. 10, no. 6, pp. 581–606, 2021.

[14] D. Joshi, S. Anwarul, and V. Mishra, "Deep learning using keras," in Mehul Mahrishi, Kamal Kant Hiran, Gaurav Meena, and Paawan Sharma (eds.), *Machine Learning and Deep Learning in Real-Time Applications*, IGI global, pp. 33–60, 2020.

[15] S. Anwarul and D. Joshi, "Deep learning with tensorflow," in Mehul Mahrishi, Kamal Kant Hiran, Gaurav Meena, and Paawan Sharma (eds.), *Machine Learning and Deep Learning in Real-Time Applications*, IGI global, pp. 96–120, 2020.

[16] I. Masi, Y. Wu, T. Hassner, and P. Natarajan, "Deep face recognition: A survey," in *2018 31st SIBGRAPI Conference on Graphics, Patterns and Images (SIBGRAPI)*, IEEE, pp. 471–478, 2018.

[17] R. Shailendra et al., "An IoT and machine learning based intelligent system for the classification of therapeutic plants," *Neural Processing Letters*, vol. 54, no. 5, pp. 4465–4493, 2022.

[18] G. Madhu et al., "DSCN-net: a deep Siamese capsule neural network model for automatic diagnosis of malaria parasites detection," *Multimedia Tools and Applications*, vol. 81, no. 23, pp. 34105–34127, 2022.

[19] L. Stark, A. Stanhaus, and D. L. Anthony, "'I don't want someone to watch me while i'm working': Gendered views of facial recognition technology in workplace surveillance," *Journal of the Association for Information Science and Technology*, vol. 71, no. 9, pp. 1074–1088, 2020.

[20] C. Tan et al., "A survey on deep transfer learning," in *Artificial Neural Networks and Machine Learning–ICANN 2018*, Springer, pp. 270–279, 2018.

[21] S. J. Pan and Q. Yang, "A survey on transfer learning," *IEEE Transactions on Knowledge and Data Engineering*, vol. 22, no. 10, pp. 1345–1359, 2010.

[22] M. A. Ganaie, M. Hu, A. K. Malik, M. Tanveer, and P. N. Suganthan, "Ensemble deep learning: A review," *Engineering Applications of Artificial Intelligence*, vol. 115, p. 105151, 2022.

[23] Starlink, "Facial Recognition Technology: Functionality, Applications, & Significance in Today's World," [Online]. Available: www.starlinkindia. com/blog/facial-recognition-technology-functionality-applications-significa nce-in-todays-world/. [Accessed: 1-May-2024].

[24] B. S. Khade, H. M. Gaikwad, A. S. Aher, and K. 3. Patil, "Face recognition techniques: a survey," *International Journal of Computer Science and Mobile Computing*, vol. 5, no. 11, pp. 65–72, 2016.

[25] T. C. Fu, W. C. Chiu, and Y. C. F. Wang, "Learning guided convolutional neural networks for cross-resolution face recognition," in *2017 IEEE 27th International Workshop on Machine Learning for Signal Processing (MLSP)*, IEEE, pp. 1–5, 2017.

[26] W. Zhang, S. Shan, X. Chen, and W. Gao, "Local Gabor binary patterns based on Kullback–Leibler divergence for partially occluded face recognition," *IEEE Signal Processing Letters*, vol. 14, no. 11, pp. 875–878, 2007.

[27] W. W. Zou and P. C. Yuen, "Very low resolution face recognition problem," *IEEE Transactions on Image Processing*, vol. 21, no. 1, pp. 327–340, 2011.

[28] H. K. K. Tin, "Removal of noise by median filtering in image processing," in *6th Parallel Soft Comput. (PSC 2011)*, University of Computer Studies, Yangon, pp. 1–3, 2011.

[29] Z. Luo, J. Hu, W. Deng, and H. Shen, "Deep unsupervised domain adaptation for face recognition," in *2018 13th IEEE International Conference on Automatic Face & Gesture Recognition (FG 2018)*, IEEE, pp. 453–457, 2018.

[30] P. Wang, W. H. Lin, K. M. Chao, and C. C. Lo, "A face recognition approach using deep reinforcement learning approach for user authentication," in *2017 IEEE 14th International Conference on e-Business Engineering (ICEBE)*, IEEE, pp. 183–188, 2017.

[31] S. Z. S. Chu, R. Liao, and L. Zhang, "Illumination invariant face recognition using near-infrared images," *IEEE Transactions on Pattern Analysis and Machine Intelligence*, vol. 29, no. 4, pp. 627–639, 2007.

[32] S. Banerjee et al., "To frontalize or not to frontalize: Do we really need elaborate pre-processing to improve face recognition?," in *2018 IEEE Winter Conference on Applications of Computer Vision (WACV)*, IEEE, pp. 20–29, 2018.

[33] Y. Gao and H. J. Lee, "Cross-pose face recognition based on multiple virtual views and alignment error," *Pattern Recognition Letters*, vol. 65, pp. 170–176, 2015.

[34] C. Ding, C. Xu, and D. Tao, "Multi-task pose-invariant face recognition," *IEEE Transactions on Image Processing*, vol. 24, no. 3, pp. 980–993, 2015.

[35] R. Singh, M. Vatsa, A. Ross, and A. Noore, "A mosaicing scheme for pose invariant face recognition," *IEEE Transactions on Systems, Man, and Cybernetics, Part B (Cybernetics)*, vol. 37, no. 5, pp. 1212–1225, 2007.

[36] T. Ahonen, A. Hadid, and M. Pietikainen, "Face description with local binary patterns: Application to face recognition," *IEEE Transactions on Pattern Analysis and Machine Intelligence*, vol. 28, no. 12, pp. 2037–2041, 2006.

[37] H. Zhou and K. M. Lam, "Age-invariant face recognition based on identity inference from appearance age," *Pattern Recognition*, vol. 76, pp. 191–202, 2018.

[38] Z. Li, U. Park, and A. K. Jain, "A discriminative model for age invariant face recognition," *IEEE Transactions on Information Forensics and Security*, vol. 6, no. 3, pp. 1028–1037, 2011.

[39] M. Mun and A. Deorankar, "Implementation of plastic surgery face recognition using multimodal biometric features," *International Journal of Computer Science and Information Technology*, vol. 5, no. 3, pp. 3711–3715, 2014.

[40] A. Mathew, P. Amudha, and S. Sivakumari, "Deep learning techniques: an overview," in *Advanced Machine Learning Technologies and Applications: Proceedings of AMLTA 2020*, Springer, pp. 599–608, 2021.

[41] A. Panigrahi, Y. Chen, and C. C. J. Kuo, "Analysis on gradient propagation in batch normalized residual networks," arXiv preprint arXiv:1812.00342, 2018.

[42] J. Lorraine and D. Duvenaud, "Stochastic hyperparameter optimization through hypernetworks," arXiv preprint arXiv:1802.09419, 2018.

[43] A. Vieira and B. Ribeiro, *Introduction to deep learning business applications for developers*. Berkeley, CA, USA: Apress, 2018.

[44] M. Lin, Q. Chen, and S. Yan, "Network in network," *Computing Research Repository (CoRR)*, vol. 1312, no. 4400, 2013.

[45] T. Takahashi, "U.S. Patent No. 10,013,644," Washington, DC: U.S. Patent and Trademark Office, 2018.

[46] N. Srivastava et al., "Dropout: A simple way to prevent neural networks from overfitting," *Journal of Machine Learning Research*, vol. 15, no. 1, pp. 1929–1958, 2014.

[47] A. Achille and S. Soatto, "Information dropout: Learning optimal representations through noisy computation," *IEEE Transactions on Pattern Analysis and Machine Intelligence*, vol. 40, no. 12, pp. 2897–2905, 2018.

[48] S. Ioffe and C. Szegedy, "Batch normalization: Accelerating deep network training by reducing internal covariate shift," in *International Conference on Machine Learning*, PMLR (Proceedings of Machine Learning Research), pp. 448–456, 2015.

[49] R. Polikar, *Ensemble machine learning: Methods and applications*. New York, NY, USA: John Wiley & Sons, Inc., 2012.

[50] "Overview of hyperparameter tuning | Vertex AI | Google Cloud," Google Cloud. [Online]. Available: https://cloud.google.com/vertex-ai/docs/train ing/hyperparameter-tuning-overview. [Accessed: 5-May-2024].

[51] "Anyscale – What is hyperparameter tuning?," Anyscale. [Online]. Available: www.anyscale.com/blog/what-is-hyperparameter-tuning. [Accessed: 10-May-2024].

[52] L. N. Smith, "Cyclical learning rates for training neural networks," In *2017 IEEE Winter Conference on Applications of Computer Vision (WACV)*, IEEE, pp. 464–472, 2017.

[53] C. Shorten and T. M. Khoshgoftaar, "A survey on image data augmentation for deep learning," *Journal of Big Data*, vol. 6, no. 1, pp. 1–48, 2019.

[54] G. B. Huang, M. Mattar, T. Berg, and E. Learned-Miller, "Labeled faces in the wild: A database for studying face recognition in unconstrained environments," In *Workshop on faces in Real-Life Images: Detection, Alignment, and Recognition*, ECCV, 2008.

Chapter 4

Neuromorphic horizons

Exploring the intersection of generative AI and brain-inspired computing in secured healthcare

Roohi Sille

4.1 INTRODUCTION

Using the structure and operations of the human brain as inspiration, neuromorphic computing is a cutting-edge method of creating computational systems. Neural processing is distributed and occurs in parallel, unlike in typical von Neumann systems, which divide processing and memory units [1]. This is the goal of neuromorphic computing.

Essentially, neuromorphic computing leverages the energy-saving, fault-tolerant, and efficient characteristics found in biological brain networks to circumvent the constraints of traditional computer paradigms. The creation of synaptic connections that facilitate learning and information processing, as well as the imitation of spiking neurons—the fundamental computational units of the brain—achieve this [2].

Event-driven computation, which mimics the asynchronous nature of neuronal activity by processing input only when substantial system changes occur, is one of the fundamental ideas of neuromorphic computing. Neuromorphic systems are well-suited for applications like edge computing, robotics, and sensor processing because of this approach's ability to operate at little power and respond instantly.

The variety of neuromorphic hardware implementations includes digital neuromorphic processors and custom-designed analogue circuits, each with its own advantages in terms of speed, scalability, and energy efficiency. Examples are the SpiNNaker project by the Human Brain Project, the Loihi chip from Intel, and the TrueNorth chip from IBM.

Beyond hardware, neuromorphic computing includes simulation tools and software frameworks for creating neuromorphic algorithms and modelling neural networks. With the aid of these instruments, scientists may investigate the dynamics of intricate neural networks and create cutting-edge learning algorithms that are motivated by biological processes [3].

All things considered, neuromorphic computing has the potential to open new vistas in the fields of artificial intelligence, neuroscience, and cognitive science by providing a means of developing more effective and brain-like

DOI: 10.1201/9781003518075-4

computer systems that can handle problems in a variety of real-world contexts.

One revolutionary area of artificial intelligence is called "generative AI," which is concerned with creating new instances of data, be they text, audio, images, or other kinds of material. To generate unique and realistic results, generative AI seeks to comprehend and mimic the underlying patterns and structures seen in a dataset, in contrast to traditional AI techniques that are superior at tasks like categorization or prediction.

Generative models, or neural networks trained to discover the underlying probability distribution of a given dataset, are the brains behind generative artificial intelligence. Then, these models can produce new samples that have unique subtleties and differences while still resembling the original data. Generative Adversarial Networks (GANs) and Variational Autoencoders (VAEs) are two popular generative model types, each having specific advantages and uses.

Introduced in 2014 by Ian Goodfellow and colleagues, GANs are composed of a generator and a discriminator neural network [4]. While the discriminator learns to discern between genuine and produced samples, the generator learns to produce realistic data samples. Generating photorealistic images and synthesizing convincing voice and music are just two examples of the many fields in which GANs can yield high-quality outputs through adversarial training, in which the generator and discriminator compete with one another.

Conversely, VAEs are probabilistic models that map input data to a lower-dimensional latent space to uncover the latent structure of the data. VAEs create samples by taking a sample from the learned latent space and decoding it back into the original data space, in contrast to GANs, which create samples through a discriminative process. VAEs are very good at capturing the underlying uncertainty and variability in the data, which makes them suitable for tasks like data denoising, representation learning, and picture production.

Recent improvements in deep learning, large-scale datasets, and computer resources have propelled the amazing progress of generative AI. Generative models have shown an unparalleled level of inventiveness and ingenuity, producing everything from lifelike human faces to unique musical compositions. Generative AI has the potential to be used in many different contexts, such as content generation, data enrichment, personalized recommendation systems, and even supporting creative and scientific endeavors.

Due to their shared objective of simulating the extraordinary capacities of the human brain, neuromorphic computing and generative AI have come together to form a promising new area in artificial intelligence research. This junction offers great potential for developing both domains and tackling important computing and AI issues.

The highlights of this chapter are as follows:

1. Thorough investigation of the application of generative AI models and neuromorphic computing, two cutting-edge technologies.
2. The GAN and neuromorphic architectures utilized in healthcare are thoroughly examined.
3. In-depth analysis of the benefits and drawbacks of computational models created with these technologies.
4. Future directions for the development of neuromorphic architectures for diagnosis and prognosis in medicine.

The chapter is structured as follows: Section I covers the issue overview, and Section II talks about the survey that was done on neuromorphic architectures that are used in medical treatment. In Section III, GAN models in healthcare are examined. The junction of the two more general categories—neuromorphic computing and GANs—is examined in Section IV. The neuromorphic methods for improving generative AI are examined in Section V, and the final section addresses conclusions and future directions.

4.2 LITERATURE SURVEY

The history and advancement of neuromorphic computers date back to the middle of the twentieth century, and they have seen substantial change since then. This is a survey conducted:

a) Early Concepts (1940s-1960s):
   The foundation of neuromorphic computing is found in the groundbreaking research of academics like Walter Pitts and Warren McCulloch, [5, 6] who in the 1940s created mathematical models of artificial neurons. The theoretical groundwork for employing computer models to simulate neural networks was established by their work. Researchers like Frank Rosenblatt created the perceptron, an early neural network architecture that could recognize basic patterns, in the 1950s and 1960s. The perceptron, despite its drawbacks, set the stage for later advances in neural network science.

b) Biological Inspiration and Parallel Processing (1970s-1980s):
   Thanks to developments in computing and neuroscience, neural network research had a renaissance in attention during the 1970s and 1980s. Scientists tried to replicate the distributed and parallel processing found in the human brain.

   The development of parallel processing architectures in computers was influenced by initiatives such as the Parallel Distributed Processing (PDP) model, which was put forth by David Rumelhart and James McClelland to investigate the computational foundations underpinning human cognition.

c)   Emergence of Spiking Neural Networks (1990s-2000s):
Spiking neural networks (SNNs) are a biologically inspired computational model that mimics the behavior and connections of individual neurons [6]. They first appeared in the 1990s. Spike timing in SNNs is used to encode information, much like in asynchronous neural activity found in biological systems. The creation of neuromorphic hardware was pioneered by scientists such as Carver Mead, who created analog circuits that emulated the functions of biological neurons. Future developments in hardware implementations of neuromorphic computing were made possible by initiatives such as Mead's "neuromorphic engineering".

d)   Advances in Hardware and Simulation Tools (2010s-present):
Neuromorphic computing saw a resurgence in attention in the 2010s due to developments in semiconductor technology and the growth of deep learning [7]. Businesses and academic institutions started creating customized hardware architectures that were designed to mimic brain networks and carry out neuromorphic algorithms.

BrainScaleS, IBM's TrueNorth chip, and the SpiNNaker project are examples of initiatives that have shown the viability of large-scale neuromorphic systems for cognitive computing and real-time brain simulation. Simulated neural circuits and software frameworks like NEST, Brian, and Nengo enabled academics to explore intricate brain-inspired algorithms by giving them strong platforms for modeling and simulating neural circuits.

4.2.1 Current trends and future directions

Current developments in hardware, software, and interdisciplinary cooperation are propelling the fast evolution of neuromorphic computing. In fields like neuromorphic artificial intelligence, robotics, and sensory processing, researchers are examining new designs, algorithms, and uses for neuromorphic systems.

Future directions in neuromorphic computing include exploring neuromorphic approaches to AI and machine learning, as well as developing more scalable and energy-efficient neuromorphic hardware and integrating neuromorphic and conventional computing systems. Growing in maturity, neuromorphic computing has the potential to address major issues in computing and artificial intelligence (AI), ranging from scalability and energy efficiency to cognitive intelligence and brain-inspired computing techniques.

Neuromorphic computing strives to develop intelligent systems that possess the effectiveness, flexibility, and resilience of biological neural networks by abiding by these fundamental ideas and concepts. These ideas

Table 4.1 Survey on Neuromorphic Computing in Medical Diagnosis and Prediction

Reference	Model	Dataset	Focus Area	Performance Metrics
[8]	NeuroCARE, uses a unique sparse spike encoder	EEG signals	Epileptic seizure Detection and prediction, arrhythmia detection and hand gesture recognition, respectively.	classification accuracy, sensitivity and F1 score, achieve 92.7, 96.7, and 85.7% for seizure prediction, arrhythmia detection and hand gesture recognition, respectively.
[9]	Deep SNN	EEG signals	Epileptic seizure detection	energy and computation-efficient
[10]	Hardware for deep network accelerators	EMG signals	Smart Healthcare by monitoring biomedical signal and processing it.	Reduced workloads for monitoring health data
[11]	Probabilistic Neural Network with Approximate Entropy	EEG signals	Epileptic seizures classification	Accuracy in generalised epilepsy detection is 90%

drive progress in computing, cognitive science, and artificial intelligence by guiding the design of neuromorphic hardware and algorithms.

4.2.2 Applications and advantages

Neuromorphic computing leverages its distinct advantages over conventional computing paradigms to offer a broad range of applications across multiple fields. The following are some major uses and benefits:

- Sensor Processing and Edge Computing: Real-time sensor data processing is a strong point for neuromorphic computing, which makes it perfect for uses like audio and picture processing, natural language processing, and sensor fusion. Its event-driven compute and low power consumption allow for effective edge processing, which lowers latency and bandwidth needs.
- Neuromorphic AI and Robotics: The development of intelligent systems and robots with real-time perception, learning, and interaction with their surroundings is made possible by neuromorphic computing. Neuromorphic algorithms can be used in autonomous navigation, object recognition, gesture recognition, and adaptive control, among other applications, to enable quick decision-making and condition adaption.

- Brain-Machine Interfaces (BMIs): The development of sophisticated BMIs that permit direct brain-to-external device communication appears promising considering neuromorphic computing. Neuromorphic BMIs can improve cognitive function, permit brain-controlled prosthetics and exoskeletons, and restore motor function by decoding neural signals in real-time and offering closed-loop feedback [12].

- Cognitive Computing and Neuromorphic AI: The development of cognitive computing systems with human-like intelligence and behavior is made possible by neuromorphic computing. Neuromorphic AI systems can carry out difficult cognitive tasks like pattern recognition, decision-making, and language processing more effectively and independently than traditional AI techniques because they emulate the parallelism, plasticity, and learning capacities of the brain [13].

- Energy-Efficient Computing: Energy efficiency is a major benefit of neuromorphic computing, which is a result of its low-power hardware implementations and event-driven design. When compared to conventional von Neumann architectures, neuromorphic systems use orders of magnitude less power, which makes them appropriate for battery-operated devices, Internet of Things applications, and sustainable computing solutions [14].

- Unsupervised Learning and Anomaly Detection: Unsupervised learning tasks—where the objective is to find underlying patterns and structures in data without explicit labels—are an area in which neuromorphic computing shines. Neuromorphic algorithms are useful for data analytics, cybersecurity, and anomaly detection because they can identify abnormalities, group data, and extract meaningful representations. Examples of these algorithms are spiking neural networks (SNNs) and self-organizing maps (SOMs).

- Neuromorphic Computing for Scientific Simulations: A unique method for mimicking intricate systems and events in research and engineering is provided by neuromorphic computing. Researchers can simulate large-scale neural networks, physical simulations, and dynamical systems more efficiently than with traditional supercomputers by utilizing the parallelism and efficiency of neuromorphic hardware. This allows for advancements in materials science, climate modeling, neuroscience, and drug discovery [15, 16].

All things considered, neuromorphic computing offers a wide range of benefits and applications in industries like artificial intelligence, robotics, healthcare, neuroscience, and scientific research. Neuromorphic technology could completely transform computers and bring in a new era of intelligent, energy-efficient, and brain-inspired systems as it develops.

4.3 EXPLORING GENERATIVE AI

4.3.1 Evolution of generative models

The quest to develop AI systems that can produce realistic and varied data samples has propelled the creation of generative models, resulting in notable advances in machine learning and AI. Below is a summary of significant turning points in the development of generative models:

Early Approaches (1950s-2000s):
The earliest examples of generative modeling were probabilistic models like Markov chains and Hidden Markov Models (HMMs), which were developed in the 1950s. The main application of these models was to create events or symbol sequences.

Researchers investigated Bayesian techniques for probabilistic modeling in the 1980s and 1990s. These techniques included graphical models and Bayesian networks, which offered a framework for reasoning under uncertainty and producing data using learned probability distributions.

Autoencoders and Restricted Boltzmann Machines (RBMs) (2000s):
Autoencoders were a popular method for unsupervised learning and data compression in the early 2000s. An encoder and a decoder network that have been taught to reconstruct input data make up autoencoders, which essentially teach the network how to represent the data in low dimensions.

In the 2000s, Geoffrey Hinton and associates developed restricted boltzmann machines (RBMs), which offered a probabilistic generative model that could learn intricate data distributions. Later advancements in deep generative modeling were built upon RBMs.

Deep Learning Revolution and Variational Autoencoders (VAEs) (2010s):
Deep learning transformed generative modeling in the 2010s by allowing deep neural networks to be trained on massive datasets. Generative models have become useful frameworks for learning complex data distributions, such as Variational Autoencoders (VAEs) and Generative Adversarial Networks (GANs).

Diederik P. Kingma and Max Welling proposed VAEs in 2013, which use autoencoder architectures in conjunction with variational inference to learn probabilistic generative models. By sampling from the learnt distribution, VAEs can produce fresh samples after learning a latent representation of the input.

Generative Adversarial Networks (GANs) (2014-present):
In 2014, Ian Goodfellow and associates introduced a unique paradigm for generative modeling based on adversarial training: Generative Adversarial

Networks, or GANs [17]. A generator and a discriminator are the two neural networks that make up a GAN. They are trained concurrently and in a competitive manner.

In a variety of domains, such as text, audio, video, and photos, GANs have shown impressive success in producing diverse, high-quality examples. They have been applied to data augmentation, super-resolution, style transfer, and image production, among other tasks.

Progressive and Conditional Generative Models (2017-present):
Progressive training methods for GANs are recent developments in generative modeling that allow to produce high-resolution pictures and films. Improved sample quality is the result of using progressive GANs to train the generator network gradually at various resolutions.

Data can be generated conditioned on attributes or labels using conditional generative models, such as Conditional GANs (cGANs) and Conditional VAEs (cVAEs). These models have applications in picture-to-image translation, text-to-image synthesis, and image modification; they allow for fine-grained control over the generated samples.

Hybrid and Ensemble Models (2020s):
The creation of hybrid and ensemble models, which integrate several generative architectures to increase sample diversity and quality, is one of the most recent developments in generative modeling. While ensemble models combine predictions from several models to provide more varied and reliable samples, hybrid models combine elements from other generative frameworks.

Furthermore, scientists are investigating novel approaches to generative modeling, such as the integration of physical priors, structured generative models, and neuro-symbolic methods for producing structured data and generative models that incorporate domain knowledge.

All things considered, the development of generative models has been marked by ongoing innovation and improvement, propelled by developments in deep learning, probabilistic modeling, and computing power. Scientific research, content development, medication discovery, and image generation are just a few of the many fields in which generative models have shown to be invaluable tools. We may anticipate more developments in AI and machine learning as generative modeling research moves forward, opening new avenues for creativity, exploration, and discovery.

4.3.2 Types of generative models (e.g., GANs, VAEs)

A class of machine learning models known as generative models is made to identify patterns in each dataset and use those patterns to create new data samples. These models can generate fresh samples with comparable properties by capturing the underlying distribution of the data. The following are a few well-known categories of generative models:

Autoencoders:
Neural network topologies called autoencoders comprise a decoder network and an encoder network. While the decoder reconstructs the original data from the latent space representation, the encoder compresses the input data into a low-dimensional representation (latent space). By sampling from the learnt latent space, autoencoders can be trained in an unsupervised way to produce fresh samples and acquire a compact representation of the input.

Variational Autoencoders (VAEs):
Variational Autoencoders (VAEs) add probabilistic modeling into the latent space, hence expanding the fundamental autoencoder architecture. By learning a probability distribution throughout the latent space, VAEs enable generational stochastic sampling. This makes it possible for VAEs to carry out operations like data synthesis, data denoising, and anomaly detection as well as to produce a variety of realistic samples.

Generative Adversarial Networks (GANs):
Two neural networks, a generator and a discriminator, are trained concurrently in a competitive manner to form Generative Adversarial Networks (GANs). While the discriminator learns to discern between produced and real samples, the generator learns to create realistic samples from random noise. GANs can produce diverse and high-quality samples in a range of domains, such as text, audio, video, and pictures, through adversarial training.

Autoregressive Models:
Autoregressive models are probabilistic models that generate data sequentially, one element at a time, conditioned on previously generated elements. Examples include Autoregressive Moving Average (ARMA) models, Autoregressive Integrated Moving Average (ARIMA) models, and more recently, autoregressive neural network architectures such as WaveNet and PixelCNN. Autoregressive models are particularly well-suited for generating sequential data such as time series, text, and audio.

Flow-Based Models:
Flow-based models use a sequence of invertible transformations, or flows, applied to a basic distribution (such as Gaussian) to parameterize the data distribution. By using inverse transformations, these models can efficiently generate samples by learning a mapping from the data space to a latent space where sampling is simple. Examples of state-of-the-art performance in picture generating jobs are Normalizing Flows, RealNVP, and Glow.

Energy-Based Models (EBMs):
The data distribution is represented by Energy-Based Models (EBMs) as an energy function, where high probability is associated with low energy. By using sampling and optimization approaches, these models can allocate high energy to created data and low energy to observed data, so enabling probabilistic sampling. Examples are Deep Boltzmann Machines (DBMs) and Restricted Boltzmann Machines (RBMs), which have been applied to image synthesis, data modeling, and anomaly detection, among other applications.

These are a few of the most common categories of generative models, each having unique advantages and uses. Advances in AI, machine learning, and data science are the result of researchers' ongoing exploration of novel generative modeling structures and methodologies.

4.3.3 Applications and use cases

Generative models have a wide range of applications across various domains, leveraging their ability to generate new data samples that resemble those from a given dataset. Here are some of the key applications and use cases of generative models:

Image Generation and Synthesis:
For producing realistic and varied images, generative models—in particular, Generative Adversarial Networks (GANs) and Variational Autoencoders (VAEs)—are frequently employed. High-resolution image generation, photorealistic image synthesis from textual descriptions, and artistic image and visual effect creation are some of the applications.

Data Augmentation:
Using generative models, datasets can be enhanced by creating additional samples with different looks, styles, or contents. Particularly in tasks like object detection, semantic segmentation, and picture classification, data augmentation enhances the generalization and robustness of machine learning models.

Anomaly Detection:
To detect anomalies, generative models like Energy-Based Models (EBMs) and Variational Autoencoders (VAEs) can be trained to understand the underlying distribution of normal data and spot departures from it. Applications include spotting fraudulent transactions, spotting manufacturing flaws in products, and spotting irregularities in sensor and medical picture data.

Content Creation and Creative AI:
The use of generative models in creative AI applications, such as producing poetry, music, storytelling, and artwork, is growing. These models allow for

the automation of creative duties and the discovery of new artistic styles by picking up patterns and styles from previously created works and producing new content with those same qualities.

Text Generation and Natural Language Processing (NLP):
Text creation and natural language processing tasks are performed using generative models, such as Recurrent Neural Networks (RNNs), Transformer models, and GPT (Generative Pre-trained Transformer) models. Language translation, text summarization, conversation creation, and content creation for chatbots and virtual assistants are a few examples of applications.

Drug Discovery and Molecular Design:
To create novel molecules with the right properties, generative models are used in drug discovery and chemical design. Compared to conventional methods, these models are more effective in exploring chemical space, producing novel chemical compounds, and optimizing drug candidates for certain targets, which speeds up the drug discovery process and helps develop new therapies.

Image-to-Image Translation:
Style transfer, image colorization, and picture super-resolution are examples of image-to-image translation tasks that are performed using generative models like Conditional Generative Adversarial Networks (cGANs) and CycleGANs. With the help of these models, one can convert images from one visual domain to another while maintaining the semantic meaning of the original image.

Medical Imaging and Healthcare:
In the fields of medical imaging and healthcare, generative models are used for tasks including image synthesis, denoising, and reconstruction. These models may simulate various medical imaging modalities, produce realistic medical images for training and validation, and help with diagnosis and therapy planning.

These examples represent just a fraction of the diverse range of applications that generative models have across various fields. With ongoing advancements in generative modelling techniques, we can expect to see further progress and utilization in artificial intelligence, machine learning, and data-driven disciplines. Within medical imaging and healthcare realms, generative models play crucial roles in tasks such as creating images, reducing noise, and reconstructing data. These models have the capability to mimic different medical imaging methods, generate lifelike medical images for training purposes, and aid in both diagnosis and treatment planning processes.

Table 4.2 Survey on GAN models for Medical Diagnosis and Prediction

Reference	Model	Focus Area	Dataset	Performance Measure
[18]	LSTM-GAN-AE	Fault diagnosis in machine health monitoring	Overall health monitoring	Accuracy=99.74%
[19]	GAN	Brain tumor segmentation	MRI scans (Brats)	Accuracy=97%
[20]	GAN	Medical image super resolution	DRIVE, STARE, Brats, CAMUS datasets	Achieves superior accuracy
[21]	MedGan	Medical image generation	demodicosis, blister, molluscum and parakerotosis datasets	Method proved effective for disease classification and lesion localization

4.4 BRIDGING NEUROMORPHIC COMPUTING AND GENERATIVE AI

Biological systems serve as the shared source of inspiration for both neuromorphic computing and generative artificial intelligence. Drawing upon principles from cognitive science and neuroscience, researchers aim to mimic the extraordinary capabilities of the human brain in creating adaptable and intelligent systems. The key biological elements that link generative AI with neuromorphic computing are as follows:

Parallel and Distributed Processing:
In biological brains, billions of neurons communicate through complex synaptic networks, processing information in a highly parallel and distributed manner. Neuromorphic computing structures mimic this distributed processing and parallelism to efficiently compute and learn across extensive neural networks. Like the collaborative nature of brain neurons, generative AI models utilize parallel processing methods to acquire knowledge and generate data in a distributed fashion.

Plasticity and Learning:
Neuromorphic computing and generative AI are fundamentally inspired by synaptic plasticity, the brain's capacity for adaptation and experience-based learning. To allow for learning and adaptability in artificial neural networks, neuromorphic algorithms include elements of synaptic plasticity, such as spike-timing-dependent plasticity (STDP). Like this, generative models pick up on patterns and structures in the data to enable them to create new samples that bear similarities to the training set.

Event-Driven Computation:
Processing in biological neurons is asynchronous and event-driven because they exchange information via distinct electrical impulses or spikes. This event-driven computing paradigm—in which computation only happens in reaction to input events or system changes—is embraced by neuromorphic computing. Event-driven processing is used by generative models, especially those that are based on spiking neural networks (SNNs), to effectively imitate brain dynamics and provide data that is highly efficient and has minimal latency.

Adaptation to Environment:
Because they can sense, learn, and react to stimuli, biological creatures exhibit great environmental adaptability. To mimic this adaptability, neuromorphic computing seeks to create intelligent systems that can sense and respond to their surroundings instantly. In a similar vein, generative AI models adjust to the properties of the incoming data, allowing them to produce realistic and contextually relevant samples that are customized for certain tasks and contexts.

Efficiency and Robustness:
Biological brains are incredibly powerful and resilient computational systems that can handle large volumes of data while using very little energy and remaining resilient against errors and noise. Neuromorphic computing designs use low-power hardware implementations, event-driven processing, sparse coding, and fault tolerance as top priorities. Similarly, generative AI models aim for robustness and efficiency, which allows them to function in real-world scenarios with constrained computational resources and scale to massive datasets.

Researchers in neuromorphic computing and generative AI are paving new paths toward the creation of intelligent and adaptive systems that rival the capacities of the human brain by adopting these biological inspiration principles. They are breaking new ground in AI, neurology, and computing through interdisciplinary innovation and collaboration, with significant ramifications for science, technology, and society.

Future developments and uses of these technologies will be shaped by the potential and problems that the nexus of generative AI and neuromorphic computing brings. The following are some major obstacles and chances:

Challenges:
Designing neuromorphic hardware designs is difficult and complex, especially for large-scale implementations. For hardware developers, achieving scalability without sacrificing real-time performance or energy efficiency is still a major problem.

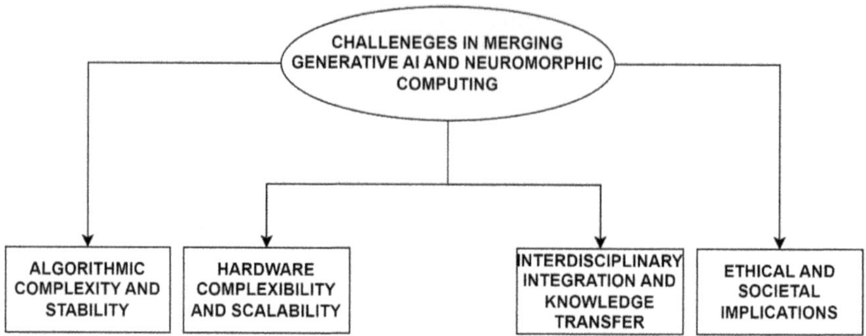

Figure 4.1 Challenges in Merging Generative AI and Neuromorphic Computing.

Particularly those based on deep neural networks, generative AI models frequently experience problems with mode collapse, convergence, and training instability. One of the main challenges in generative modeling is creating reliable training algorithms and regularization strategies to enhance stability and convergence.

Bridging the gap between neuroscience, computer science, and engineering disciplines requires interdisciplinary collaboration and knowledge transfer. Integrating insights from neuroscience into neuromorphic algorithms and architectures, while leveraging advances in machine learning and computational neuroscience, presents challenges in terms of communication, terminology, and methodology. Figure 4.1 shows challenges in Generative AI and Neuromorphic Computing.

Concerns about privacy, bias, accountability, and autonomous decision-making are among the ethical and societal issues brought up by the research and application of neuromorphic computing and generative AI. It is necessary to carefully analyze ethical standards, legal frameworks, and openness in the creation and application of AI to allay these worries.

Opportunities:
With the help of neuromorphic computing, effective and flexible computer systems modeled after the structure of the human brain may be possible. These systems enable novel applications in edge computing, robotics, and IoT since they can carry out complicated cognitive tasks with minimal power consumption and real-time response.

The development of original and imaginative content in a variety of fields, such as music, literature, design, and the arts, is made possible by generative AI models. These models have the potential to enhance human creativity, promote artistic expression, and produce innovative, entertaining,

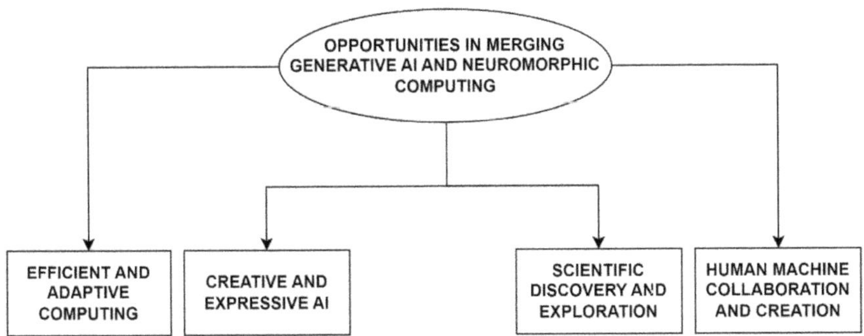

Figure 4.2 Opportunities in Merging Generative AI and Neuromorphic Computing.

and inspiring content. Figure 4.2 reveals some of the opportunities in merging generative AI and neuromorphic computing.

Personalized and adaptable user interfaces that anticipate user preferences, adjust to user behavior, and offer customized advice and support can be created using neuromorphic computing and generative artificial intelligence. These interfaces improve productivity and user experience in a variety of applications, including gaming, virtual assistants, and tailored medicine.

Accelerating scientific research and exploration in domains like neurology, drug development, materials science, and climate modelling is possible with the help of neuromorphic computers and generative AI. These technological advancements make it possible to simulate, analyze, and optimize complicated systems and phenomena, which opens new avenues for understanding and solving the world's most pressing problems.

All things considered, the difficulties and possibilities that arise from the convergence of generative AI and neuromorphic computing highlight how revolutionary these technologies have the potential to be in the ways that humans compute, create, and engage with intelligent systems in the future. Through tackling these obstacles and seizing these chances, scientists and professionals can open new directions in artificial intelligence, neurology, and computing, resulting in advancements that will benefit society.

4.5 NEUROMORPHIC APPROACHES TO ENHANCING GENERATIVE AI

4.5.1 Leveraging spiking neural networks

For several reasons, using spiking neural networks (SNNs) in neuromorphic techniques to improve generative AI shows great promise.

Biological Plausibility: Compared to conventional artificial neural networks (ANNs), SNNs more closely resemble the spiking behavior of biological neurons, which may make them better at capturing the subtleties of biological neural processing.

Efficiency: Due to its ability to simulate the behavior of biological neurons more precisely by only requiring computing when a neuron fires, spiking neural networks have the potential to be more computationally efficient, especially in terms of power consumption. In contexts where resources are limited, such edge devices or Internet of Things devices, this efficiency is essential for implementing AI.

Temporal Processing: SNNs' spiking nature means that they naturally record temporal information. Due to its ability to process temporal information, SNNs are more suited for tasks like speech recognition, video analysis, and sequential decision-making. They can also more effectively represent sequences and time-series data.

Event-Driven Processing: Inspired by the brain's efficient use of resources, neuromorphic hardware functions in an event-driven fashion, meaning processing is initiated only when there is a significant change in the input. Processing is made more efficient by the event-driven paradigm's compatibility with the irregular and asynchronous character of real-world data.

Adaptability and Plasticity: Spike-timing-dependent plasticity (STDP) is one of the several types of synaptic plasticity that SNNs can display. This allows them to adapt to new information and learn from it without supervision. For generative AI jobs, where the model must learn and produce complex patterns from data, this adaptability is essential.

Nevertheless, there are still issues to be resolved, such as creating effective SNN learning algorithms, enhancing hardware implementations for real-time processing, and comprehending the dynamics of massive SNNs. Notwithstanding these difficulties, generative AI, neuromorphic hardware, and spiking neural networks have a lot to offer in terms of improving our comprehension of biological intelligence and the potential of artificial intelligence systems.

4.5.2 Neuromorphic hardware acceleration for generative models

Combining the strength of generative AI with the economy of neuromorphic computing, neuromorphic hardware acceleration presents a viable path for improving the performance of generative models. There is a great deal of promise in this convergence for the fields of drug discovery, natural language processing, and image production. The following are some advantages of neuromorphic hardware acceleration for generative models:

1. Energy Efficiency: Designed to resemble the neural networks found in the brain, neuromorphic hardware architectures provide significant energy savings over standard computers. With neuromorphic hardware for generative models, we may make significant gains in energy efficiency, allowing for more economical and environmentally friendly model deployment and training.

2. Real-time Inference: Real-time inference for generative models is made possible by the superior parallel processing and reduced latency operations of neuromorphic technology. This feature is especially helpful for situations where quick decision-making and responsiveness are essential, like video production.

3. Biological Plausibility: Generative models can function in a more biologically plausible way thanks to neuromorphic hardware architectures, which closely mimic the neuronal structure and dynamics of the brain. As a result, a variety of activities, such as voice and picture synthesis, may perform better and produce more realistic results.

4. Scalability: Large-scale generative models may be deployed effectively thanks to the intrinsic scalability of neuromorphic technology. We can train and use increasingly powerful generative models that can handle big datasets and challenging tasks by utilizing the parallelism and flexibility of neuromorphic architectures.

5. Adaptive Learning: Adaptive learning processes are supported by neuromorphic technology, which allows generative models to continually improve and adjust to changing contexts. Applications like anomaly detection and adaptive control systems, where the distribution of data varies over time, greatly benefit from this capability.

6. Low-latency Feedback Loops: Real-time interaction and adaptability can be facilitated by neuromorphic technology through low-latency feedback loops between generative models and sensory inputs. This is especially important for applications like autonomous systems and robotics, where prompt reactions to external cues are crucial.

7. Privacy-preserving Computing: For privacy-preserving computing, neuromorphic hardware can be used to enable generative models to produce outputs without disclosing private information. Neuromorphic hardware reduces privacy issues related to centralized data processing by directly executing calculations on encrypted data.

Finally, neuromorphic hardware acceleration presents a great deal of promise for generative models, providing gains in low-latency feedback loops, scalability, biological plausibility, energy efficiency, real-time inference, adaptive learning, and privacy-preserving computing. We should anticipate seeing more complex and adaptable generative AI systems powered by neuromorphic hardware acceleration as this field of study and development continues to advance.

Neuromorphic-inspired Learning Algorithms
The form and operation of biological neural networks serve as an inspiration for neuromorphic-inspired learning algorithms, which seek to emulate the effectiveness, flexibility, and resilience of these systems in artificial environments. In neuromorphic hardware architectures, these algorithms make use of concepts like sparsity, event-driven processing, and synaptic plasticity to facilitate learning and inference [6, 7]. Here are some instances of learning algorithms that draw inspiration from neuromorphics:

1. **Spiking Neural Networks (SNNs)**: Artificial neural networks (ANNs) function by means of spikes, which are distinct bursts of activity that resemble the firing of brain neurons. Spike-timing-dependent plasticity (STDP), a learning rule that adjusts synaptic connection strength based on the relative timing of pre- and post-synaptic spikes, is a common component of neuromorphic-inspired learning algorithms for SNNs. SNNs can learn temporal patterns and carry out tasks like event-based recognition and classification thanks to STDP.

2. **Unsupervised Learning**: Hebbian learning and competitive learning are two examples of neuromorphic-inspired unsupervised learning algorithms that look for patterns and structure in data without the need for explicit supervision. Hebbian learning facilitates the development of coherent memories by fortifying synaptic connections between neurons that are activated at the same time. Conversely, competitive learning drives neurons to fight for activation in response to input, which results in the formation of unique clusters or feature detectors.

3. **Reinforcement Learning**: Reinforcement learning algorithms that are inspired by neuromorphics integrate concepts from machine learning and neurology to allow agents to interact with their surroundings and learn the best course of action. Neuromorphic-inspired elements, including eligibility traces, which record the past of current events and affect learning over time, are frequently incorporated into these algorithms. In neuromorphic systems, reinforcement learning can result in effective and flexible control schemes for autonomous vehicles, video games, and robots.

4. **Event-based Processing**: The asynchronous, low-power characteristics of neuromorphic hardware are leveraged by neuromorphic-inspired learning algorithms for event-based processing to provide effective and real-time computation. Incoming sensory data is frequently processed by these algorithms on an

event-by-event basis, utilizing learning mechanisms that modify synaptic weights in reaction to external spikes. Because neuromorphic systems can process information in a highly parallel and energy-efficient manner thanks to event-based learning, they are well-suited for tasks like gesture recognition, object tracking, and sensor fusion.

5. **Neuromodulation**: Learning algorithms that draw inspiration from neuromorphic structures could integrate neuromodulatory mechanisms, which dynamically adjust the learning process according to the internal and external conditions of the body. Neuromorphic systems can adjust to shifting task demands and environmental variables through the influence of neuromodulation on synaptic plasticity, neuronal excitability, and network dynamics. Neuromodulatory learning algorithms allow artificial systems to behave in a flexible and context-sensitive manner, like how biological creatures can adapt.

To summarize, learning algorithms that are inspired by neuromorphic systems utilize brain principles to provide effective, flexible, and resilient learning inside synthetic environments. These algorithms confer great efficiency and flexibility to neuromorphic hardware architectures by utilizing spiking neural networks, unsupervised learning mechanisms, reinforcement learning techniques, event-based processing, and neuromodulatory mechanisms to perform a wide range of cognitive tasks.

4.6 FUTURE DIRECTIONS AND CHALLENGES

While combining generative AI and neuromorphic computing has enormous potential, there are several obstacles to overcome. The following are some problems and potential directions for this integration:

Enhanced Efficiency: One of the main objectives is to use neuromorphic computing's capacity to imitate the neural architecture of the brain to increase the effectiveness of generative AI algorithms. This may result in training and inference procedures that are quicker and use less energy.

Biological Plausibility: Unlike conventional computing, neuromorphic computing seeks to mimic the composition and operations of the brain more precisely. To help generative AI systems learn and provide more lifelike results, future directions entail improving neuromorphic models to more closely mimic biological processes.

Scalability: One major problem is scaling up neuromorphic computing systems to address the complexity of large-scale generative AI activities. To effectively manage the growing demands of generative AI applications, future research must concentrate on creating scalable systems and algorithms.

Robustness and Generalization: Neuromorphic computing-trained generative AI models must be durable and able to generalize across different tasks and datasets. Deploying these systems in real-world contexts requires addressing overfitting, bias, and adversarial attack concerns.

Interpretability and Explainability: Ensuring the interpretability and openness of generative AI systems' outputs is crucial, particularly for vital applications like autonomous cars and healthcare, as these systems grow more sophisticated. Future work will focus on creating explanations for the decision-making and output-generating processes of neuromorphic-based generative models.

Hardware Advancements: To fully realize the promise of this integration, memristors and neuromorphic chips—two types of neuromorphic hardware—must progress. Creating innovative hardware architectures that can effectively enable the training and inference of generative AI models is one of the future paths to pursue.

Ethical and Social Implications: Concerns about ethics and society are raised by the combination of generative AI and neuromorphic computing, as with any new technology. Future studies should investigate topics like algorithmic prejudice, data privacy, and the effects of AI-generated content on society.

Cross-disciplinary Collaboration: Collaboration between several academic fields, including neurology, computer science, engineering, and ethics, is necessary to address the difficulties and realize the potential of combining neuromorphic computing and generative AI. To properly address these intricate issues, future approaches in research will include promoting interdisciplinary efforts.

Integrating neuromorphic computing with generative AI could result in ground-breaking improvements in AI-driven creativity, problem-solving, and human-machine interaction by tackling these issues and investigating novel approaches.

4.7 CONCLUSION

In summary, the fusion of generative AI and neuromorphic computing is a cutting edge that will have a significant impact on artificial intelligence, neurology, and society. Neuromorphic computing is a promising method to improve the effectiveness, adaptability, and biological plausibility of generative AI systems by imitating the structure and operations of the brain. This merging will eventually improve the medical diagnosis and prognosis by accurately monitoring the health, classifying the disease and simultaneously predicting the diseases.

Scalability, robustness, interpretability, and ethical issues should be resolved to fully utilize this integration. The researchers of this field should individually analyze the emergence model of neuromorphic architectures and GAN to accelerate towards secured healthcare environments and provide the most accurate and precise health monitoring.

The major challenges faced in integration of GAN and neuromorphic computing for secured healthcare is high end hardware architecture to import generative AI that can handle large amount of healthcare data. It's tough to analyse the large scans of medical images through which the complete analysis of the body is possible. Integration also benefits in faster computational processing of the big data of medical scans, electronic health record, etc.

REFERENCES

1. Keerthika, R., & Abinayaa, M. S. (Eds.). (2022). *Algorithms of Intelligence: Exploring the World of Machine Learning*. Inkbound Publishers.
2. Isik, M., Vishwamith, H., Inadagbo, K., & Dikmen, I. (2023). HPCNeuroNet: Advancing Neuromorphic Audio Signal Processing with Transformer-Enhanced Spiking Neural Networks. *arXiv preprint arXiv:2311.12449*.
3. Bielza, C., & Larrañaga, P. (2020). *Data-driven computational neuroscience: machine learning and statistical models*. Cambridge University Press.
4. Goodfellow, I., Pouget-Abadie, J., Mirza, M., Xu, B., Warde-Farley, D., Ozair, S., ... & Bengio, Y. (2020). Generative adversarial networks. *Communications of the ACM, 63*(11), 139–144.
5. Abraham, T. H. (2002). (Physio) logical circuits: The intellectual origins of the McCulloch–Pitts neural networks. *Journal of the History of the Behavioral Sciences, 38*(1), 3–25.
6. Su, F., Liu, C., & Stratigopoulos, H. G. (2023). Testability and dependability of AI hardware: Survey, trends, challenges, and perspectives. *IEEE Design & Test, 40*(2), 8–58.
7. Petrovici, M. A. (2024, Apr). The coming decade of digital brain research- A vision for neuroscience at the intersection of technology and computing. *Imaging Neuroscience, 2.*
8. Tian, F., Yang, J., Zhao, S., & Sawan, M. (2023). NeuroCARE: A generic neuromorphic edge computing framework for healthcare applications. *Frontiers in Neuroscience, 17*, 1093865.
9. Zarrin, P. S., Zimmer, R., Wenger, C., & Masquelier, T. (2020). Epileptic seizure detection using a neuromorphic-compatible deep spiking neural network. In *Bioinformatics and Biomedical Engineering: 8th International Work-Conference, IWBBIO 2020, Granada, Spain, May 6–8, 2020, Proceedings 8* (pp. 389–394). Springer International Publishing.
10. Azghadi, M. R., Lammie, C., Eshraghian, J. K., Payvand, M., Donati, E., Linares-Barranco, B., & Indiveri, G. (2020). Hardware implementation of deep network accelerators towards healthcare and biomedical applications. *IEEE Transactions on Biomedical Circuits and Systems, 14*(6), 1138–1159.
11. Sharma, G., & Pradhan, N. (2012). Implementation of probabilistic neural network using approximate entropy to detect epileptic seizures. *Undergraduate Academic Research Journal, 1*(1). Article 4. DOI: 10.47893/UARJ.2012.1003
12. Fares, H., Ronchini, M., Zamani, M., Farkhani, H., & Moradi, F. (2022). In the realm of hybrid Brain: Human Brain and AI. *arXiv preprint arXiv:2210.01461*.

13. Amunts, K., Axer, M., Banerjee, S., Bitsch, L., Bjaalie, J. G., Brauner, P., ... & Zaborszky, L. (2024). The coming decade of digital brain research: A vision for neuroscience at the intersection of technology and computing. *Imaging Neuroscience, 2*, 1–35.

14. Oneto, L., Bunte, K., & Sperduti, A. (2020). Advances in artificial neural networks, machine learning and computational intelligence. *Neurocomputing, 416*, 172–176.

15. Hofmann, P., Rückel, T., & Urbach, N. (2021). Innovating with artificial intelligence: capturing the constructive functional capabilities of deep generative learning. *Proceedings of the Annual Hawaii International Conference on System Sciences*, 2021. doi:10.24251/hicss.2021.669

16. Furber, S. (2016). Large-scale neuromorphic computing systems. *Journal of Neural Engineering, 13*(5), 051001. DOI: 10.1088/1741-2560/13/5/051001

17. Merolla, P. A., Arthur, J. V., Alvarez-Icaza, R., Cassidy, A. S., Sawada, J., Akopyan, F., ... & Modha, D. S. (2014). A million spiking-neuron integrated circuit with a scalable communication network and interface. *Science, 345*(6197),668–673. DOI: 10.1126/science.1254642

18. Liu, H., Zhao, H., Wang, J., Yuan, S., & Feng, W. (2021). LSTM-GAN-AE: A promising approach for fault diagnosis in machine health monitoring. *IEEE Transactions on Instrumentation and Measurement, 71*, 1–13.

19. Sille, R., Choudhury, T., Sharma, A., Chauhan, P., Tomar, R., & Sharma, D. (2023). A novel generative adversarial network-based approach for automated brain tumour segmentation. *Medicina, 59*(1), 119.

20. Ahmad, W., Ali, H., Shah, Z., & Azmat, S. (2022). A new generative adversarial network for medical images super resolution. *Scientific Reports, 12*(1), 9533.

21. Guo, K., Chen, J., Qiu, T., Guo, S., Luo, T., Chen, T., & Ren, S. (2023). MedGAN: An adaptive GAN approach for medical image generation. *Computers in Biology and Medicine, 163*, 107119.

Chapter 5

Improving pneumonia diagnosis correctness with the synergistic approach using swin transformer and deep learning architectures on chest X-ray images

Prabal Pratap Singh, Mamta Kumari, Anubhav Dubey, Ramnayan Mishra, Prachi Chhabra, and Sunil Kumar

5.1 INTRODUCTION

Pneumonia is a grave and sometimes lethal pulmonary infection that impacts the respiratory system. A diverse array of microorganisms, including bacteria, viruses, and fungi, cause this disorder, known as respiratory infection. It can manifest with various symptoms, such as coughing, fever, and difficulty breathing [1]. Recognized as one of the deadliest infectious diseases worldwide, pneumonia ranks as the fourth leading cause of death, making it a major public health issue [2].

The diagnosis of pneumonia typically entails chest X-ray imaging, which allows for the visualization of the lungs and the identification of indications of inflammation and fluid buildup [3]. But it can be hard to tell the difference between normal and pneumonia X-rays because normal images usually show clear and see-through lung tissue, while pneumonia X-rays may show areas of opacity, fluid buildup, and inflammation [4]. Figure 5.1 presents the instances of the normal and pneumonia X-ray.

Medical professionals play a crucial role in administering the healthcare system. However, they often need extra staff, resources, and support systems to accomplish activities that are beyond their main areas of competence, such as operating complicated technology systems [5]. Within this particular framework, the incorporation of multidisciplinary domains has gained significant importance in offering innovative solutions to practical issues. A new method in the realm of medical diagnostics is the utilization of DL, a sub-part of artificial intelligence (AI) [6].

CNNs, or convolutional neural networks is sub-field of DL, and its prominent architecture like EfficientNet-B0, VGG16, VGG19, and ResNet101 has shown effectiveness at medical image classification, like chest X-rays to find pneumonia. Extensive datasets of labeled X-ray pictures can teach these algorithms, enabling them to learn the visual characteristics that indicate pneumonia. They can then evaluate new scans and make precise predictions

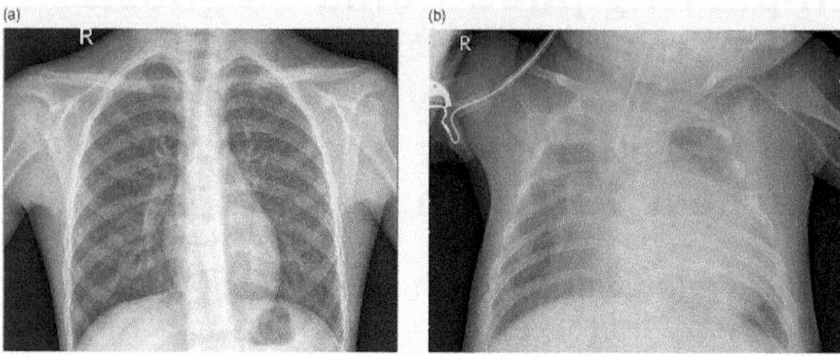

Figure 5.1 X-Ray's Instances for (a) normal and (b) pneumonia [4].

about the disease's presence [7]. This method has the capacity to enhance the velocity and precision of pneumonia diagnosis while also diminishing the burden on radiologists. Nevertheless, it is imperative to extensively evaluate these DL models on varied datasets prior to their secure use in clinical environments [8].

The Swin-T is a state-of-the-art VIT that has demonstrated superior performance on various image analysis task [9]. The proposed pneumonia detection ensemble technique uses the Swin-T as feature extractors and DL architecture for classification. Pre-training on the huge ImageNet dataset is followed by fine-tuning on the pneumonia X-ray dataset. The Swin-T is a sophisticated vision transformer that goes through each of these processes separately. The features that are obtained from the final pooling layer are used as inputs to the classification DL model. The Swin-T's exceptional ability to capture intricate and hierarchical visual representations is vital for medical image processing applications such as pneumonia identification [10, 11].

We employ the DL models to accurately classify X-ray pictures after feature extraction done by Swin-T into either pneumonia or normal categories. The models have been trained using the ImageNet dataset, and then they have been fine-tuned using the pneumonia X-ray dataset after they have been finished. The ensemble method takes the predictions made by the Swin-T feature extractor and the DL models and puts them all together. If the model produces identical predictions, the model with the highest confidence selects the final forecast. The model with higher confidence selects the final forecast if there is a disagreement. The ensemble method leverages the complementary strengths of the two models to mitigate the impact of each model's biases or limitations, thereby enhancing the resilience and generalizability of the pneumonia classification [12, 13].

This study seeks to investigate the capacity of DL approaches for diagnosing pneumonia using chest X-ray pictures. The study also aims to explore the challenges and considerations that need to be considered when developing and implementing these systems for the healthcare industry.

5.2 RELATED WORK

The detection of pneumonia on X-rays has been extensively studied, with research focusing on both DL and Swin-T techniques.

The research used 12 already-trained models trained on ImageNet to distinguish between normal x-rays and those exhibiting indications of pneumonia caused by viral or bacterial origins. Each model was assessed using standard classification measures, like accuracy and the F1 score. The majority of designs demonstrated significant performance, achieving an average f1-score of up to 84.46% when distinguishing between indicated categories. This method aids in distinguishing between typical and pneumonia-associated radiographs [7]. The research used a publicly available dataset named "Chest X-Ray Pneumonia," consisting of 5,856 AP CXRs (anteroposterior chest X-rays) from 1,583 healthy individuals and 4,273 cases of viral and bacterial pneumonia. The performance of CNN was constant across all five datasets with different amounts of noise. The standard datasets achieved an accuracy rate of 90.2%, a specificity rate of 76.1%, and a sensitivity rate of 98.7% [8]. The proposed fusion approach combines the capabilities of DL with the transformer encoder. DenseNet201, InceptionResNetV2, and Xception are the components that make up Ensemble B. On the other hand, Ensemble Model A is a combination of DenseNet201, VGG16, and GoogleNet. The foundation makes use of two different approaches in order to extract significant features from X-ray pictures, while the transformer encoder makes use of the MLP self-attention mechanism in order to guarantee an accurate diagnosis [12]. The Kermany [14] and RSNA [15] datasets didn't have a lot of data, so the researchers used deep transfer learning to combine three DL models: GoogLeNet, ResNet-18, and DenseNet-121. Their approach involved using an average ensembling strategy, where they combined the weights of state-of-the-art base learners. The analysis revealed that, in some cases, the ensemble structure faced difficulties in generating dependable projections [16]. The experiment utilized transfer learning approaches with pre-trained CNN models, such as DenseNet, VGGNet, and EfficientNet, trained on ImageNet. The data was preprocessed using CLAHE (contrast-limited adaptive histogram equalization) and BEASF (bi-histogram equalization) using the Adaptive Sigmoid Function. Expanding the dataset for analysis will increase its size, and evaluating the diagnostic system using fewer performance criteria will also help. Enhancements are necessary for certain CNN systems to enable accurate decision-making, given their provision of erroneous predictions [17]. The Condorcet's Jury Theorem (CJT) is a distinctive approach that calculates vote scores for ensemble classifiers. Using CJT, models within the voter pool could improve the accuracy of determining the majority. The performance of a CJT-based ensemble classification system was compared to that of a distinctive domain extended transfer learning (DETL) ensemble learner utilizing a soft voting ensemble. The objective was to discover whether the approach yielded superior results [18]. DenseNet169, MobileNetV2, and ViT are pre-trained convolutional neural network models that have undergone fine-tuning specifically for the project. The results are obtained by combining the extracted characteristics from the three models during the experimental stage and then performing classification [19]. PneuNet, a technique based on Vision Transformer (VIT), employs channel-based attention for image diagnosis. It applies multi-head attention to channel patches rather than feature patches. Nevertheless, the distribution of the dataset, which has the potential to introduce biases, is non-standard [20].

5.3 MATERIAL AND METHODS

Here is a detailed methodology section for the pneumonia detection using an ensemble method with Swin-T and DL architectures:

5.3.1 Dataset

The X-ray depictions utilized were acquired through participation in a Kaggle challenge, which is a publicly available dataset of X-ray scan images for the detection of pneumonia. The competition comprised a grand total of 5,863 chest X-ray scans, encompassing individuals diagnosed with pneumonia as well as those in good condition [4, 14]. During our inquiry, we evaluated X-ray scans with the intention of utilizing 80% of them for training and 20% for testing.

5.3.2 Preprocessing

Prior to training the models, the initial data sets revealed many concerns that required additional examination. The dataset was preprocessed in the following manner:

1. Resizing: The training picture for machine learning models must possess identical dimensions to the raw images, as the latter are available in diverse sizes. The images in the dataset have a spatial resolution of [224 x 224] pixels and are stored in the jpeg format. All images were resized to a consistent size of 224x224 pixels to match the input requirements of the DL architectures [21].

2. Scaling: Rapid image scaling is necessary in order to prepare for DL models. The pixel values are represented as 8-bit grayscale intensities, ranging from 0 (black) to 255 (white). The pixel values were then normalized to the range of 0 to 1 by dividing each pixel value by 255 [22].

3. Data Augmentation: To increase the diversity of the training data and improve the model's generalization capabilities, the following data augmentation techniques were applied:
    *   Random Rotation: Each image was randomly rotated by an angle between -20 and 20 degrees.
    *   Horizontal Flipping: Each image had a 50% chance of being horizontally flipped.
    *   Brightness Adjustment: The brightness of each image was randomly adjusted by a factor between 0.8 and 1.2 [23].

The preprocessed dataset was then split into training, validation, and test sets using a stratified sampling approach to ensure a balanced representation of pneumonia and normal cases in each subset.

5.3.3 Ensemble method

An ensemble method is utilized to enhance the performance of the pneumonia detection system. An average vote strategy was used to integrate the predictions from the Swin-T feature extractor and the DL architectures.

The suggested ensemble technique for pneumonia identification utilizes the synergistic advantages of the Swin-T [9] and DL architectures [12]. Initially, the Swin-T, an advanced VIT, is utilized as the feature extractor. Following preliminary training on the comprehensive ImageNet a database, the Swin-T model was refined using the pneumonia X-ray dataset. During the process of fine-tuning, the initial layers of the Swin-T were kept unchanged to maintain their ability to extract generic visual features, but the latter layers were adjusted to focus only on the objective of detecting pneumonia. The characteristics derived from the ultimate pooling layer of the refined Swin-T model were subsequently employed as inputs for the classification model. The Swin-T is chosen as the feature extractor due to its exceptional ability to capture intricate and hierarchical visual representations that are crucial for medical image analysis applications, such as pneumonia identification [9, 10]. Subsequently, the features retrieved from the Swin-T are input into the DL architecture to ultimately classify the X-ray pictures as either pneumonia or normal (healthy). DL architectures such as EfficientNet-B0, VGG16, VGG19, and ResNet101 are compact and effective CNNs that have showcased cutting-edge performance on diverse image classification assignments, including the analysis of medical images [12]. During fine-tuning, the initial layers were kept unchanged, while the later layers were modified to take advantage of the generic visual feature extraction skills. The ensemble method aggregates the predictions generated by the Swin-T feature extractor and the DL architectures through a majority voting strategy. If an ensemble model makes an identical prediction, the class that they forecast is chosen as the ultimate prediction. If there is a disagreement, the forecast is made based on the model with higher confidence, which is defined by the output probability of the model. The reason for utilizing an ensemble method is to take advantage of the complementary strengths of the two models and minimize the influence of individual model biases or weaknesses. This leads to an enhancement in the overall resilience and generality of the pneumonia detection system [9–12].

The reason for utilizing an ensemble method is to use the complementary strengths of the two models and minimize the influence of individual model biases or weaknesses, thereby enhancing the overall resilience and generalizability of the pneumonia detection system.

5.3.4 Feature extraction using Swin-T

The Swin-T model was used as the feature extractor in the proposed ensemble method. The Swin-T is a state-of-the-art VIT that has demonstrated superior performance on various image analysis tasks, including medical image analysis. The pre-trained Swin-T model was fine-tuned on the employed pneumonia X-ray dataset. Throughout the tuning process, the weights of earlier layers were stationary, and merely the weights of the later layers were updated to preserve the general visual feature extraction capabilities learned on the large-scale ImageNet dataset. The features extracted from the final pooling layer of the fine-tuned Swin-T model were then used as inputs to the DL classification model [9, 12].

- **Remove Top Layers:** In the first phase of the process, the top layers of the Swin-T model, which are in charge of feature extraction, are eliminated. This is due to the fact that we are interested in making use of the lower-level properties that learning layers have acquired.
- **Feature Extraction:** The results of the Swin-T model's last layer are then input into a feature extraction pipeline once they have been processed successfully. This pipeline consists of flattening the output of the convolutional layer into a 1D vector and feeding it into a feature extractor function [11].

The pivotal equation within the Swin-T pertains to the self-attention mechanism, which enables the model to discern input data dependencies spanning extensive distances. The equation representing self-attention in Swin-T is as follows:

$$Attention(Q,K,V) = softmax\left(\frac{(Q*K^T)}{\sqrt{d_k}}\right)*V \tag{1}$$

Where:

Q is stands for Query, is a matrix representing the query vectors, acquired through the linear projection of the input features.

K is stands for Key, is a matrix representing the key vectors, also acquired through the linear projection of the input features.

V is stands for Value, is a matrix representing the value vectors, acquired through the linear projection of the input features.

d_k is the dimension of the key vectors.

The self-attention mechanism in the Swin-T model enables it to efficiently acquire distant relationships and overall information in the input data, which is essential for applications like as picture categorization [9].

5.3.5 Classification using deep learning architecture

The features extracted by the Swin-T were fed into an DL architecture like VGG16, VGG19 [24], ResNet101 [25], and EfficientNet-B0 [26] for the final classification of the X-ray images into pneumonia or normal (healthy) classes. The DL architecture is a lightweight and efficient convolutional neural network that has achieved state-of-the-art performance on various image classification tasks, including medical image analysis. The specified DL architecture was also pre-trained on the ImageNet dataset and fine-tuned on the pneumonia X-ray dataset. Throughout the tuning process, the weights of the earlier layers were stationary, and only the weights of the later layers were updated to leverage the general visual feature extraction capabilities learned on the large-scale ImageNet dataset [9–12].

5.3.6 Performance metrics

In the context of image classification tasks, a variety of evaluation metrics are commonly used to assess the performance of DL models. Accuracy is a fundamental metric that measures the overall proportion of correctly classified instances. Precision focuses on the model's ability to avoid false positives, quantifying how many of the predicted positive instances are truly positive. Recall, or sensitivity, evaluates the model's capability to identify all the true positive instances [21]. The F1-score is a harmonic mean of precision and recall, providing a balanced measure that considers both type I and type II errors. These complementary metrics offer insights into different aspects of model performance, allowing researchers and practitioners to thoroughly evaluate the strengths and weaknesses of their DL-based image classification systems. By carefully considering these evaluation metrics, developers can make informed decisions and iteratively improve their models to achieve optimal performance for the given task and dataset [22].

5.4 RESULTS AND DISCUSSION

The examination aimed to contrast the performance of applied DL architectures on the task of diagnosing pneumonia using the Paul Mooney dataset from Kaggle. To conduct the research, the Paul Mooney dataset was employed, which contains 5,863 images of the chest X-ray. The dataset was preprocessed and split into training and test sets, maintaining the balance between pneumonia and normal cases. Each image was labeled as either normal or pneumonia. The architectures tested were ResNet-101, EfficientNet-B0, VGG16, and VGG19.

The images were preprocessed by resizing to 224x224 pixels and normalizing. Image normalization is a technique used to standardize the pixel values of an image, ensuring that all images have the same scale and range of values. This is important for the image analysis task, as it can improve the performance and accuracy of DL architectures.

The images were then input to the Swin-T for extracting relevant extracted features, which were further processed and standardized before being fed into the DL architectures ResNet-101, EfficientNet-B0, VGG16, and VGG19. The extracted features were then used as input for each DL architecture. Feature extraction is an important step that involves extracting relevant information or features from an X-ray image. VGG16 is a deep CNN that was trained on the ImageNet dataset and is known for its ability to extract high-level features. ResNet101, on the other hand, uses residual connections to improve the training of the models, making it particularly effective for image recognition tasks.

The results presented in this study demonstrate the efficacy of combining various DL architectures like ResNet-101, EfficientNet-B0, VGG16, and VGG19 with the Swin Transformer (Swin-T) model for the specified task (Figure 5.2). Additionally, the study's results indicate that DL architectures demonstrate notable efficacy in the diagnosis of pneumonia when features are extracted from Swin-T.

The EfficientNet-B0 + Swin-T model achieved the highest overall performance, with an accuracy of 96.51%, precision of 92.98%, recall of 95.04%, and F1-score of 94.01%. This indicates that the EfficientNet-B0 backbone, when combined with the Swin-T transformer, is able to effectively capture both local and global image features, leading to robust and accurate image classification.

The ResNet-101 + Swin-T model also demonstrated strong performance, with an accuracy of 92.24%, precision of 89.8%, recall of 90.3%, and F1-score of 90.02%. The ResNet-101 architecture's ability to extract

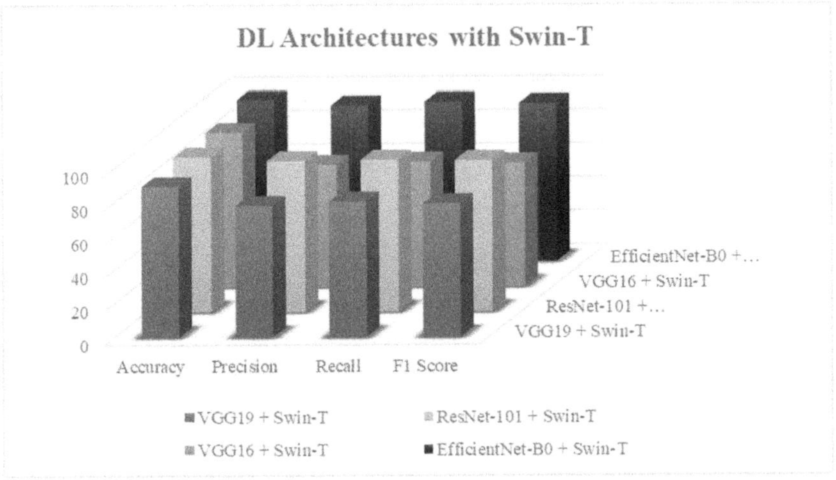

Figure 5.2 Shows the accuracy and loss for using extracted.

hierarchical features, coupled with the Swin-T model's attention-based mechanism, resulted in a highly effective classification system.

While the VGG16 + Swin-T and VGG19 + Swin-T models performed slightly worse than the ResNet-101 + Swin-T and EfficientNet-B0 + Swin-T configurations, they still achieved respectable results, with accuracies of 91.81% and 89.53%, respectively. This suggests that the VGG architectures can also benefit from integration with the Swin-T transformer, though the performance gains may be less pronounced compared to the other examined models.

The results highlight the importance of model selection and architecture combination when designing effective DL-based image classification systems. By leveraging the complementary strengths of different DL models and the Swin-T transformer, researchers and practitioners can achieve state-of-the-art performance on a variety of image recognition tasks.

However, the effectiveness of all the architectures suggests that the choice of DL architectures with Swin-T is the most critical factor in achieving an accurate pneumonia diagnosis. Instead, the eminence of the features by Swin-T and the preprocessing steps may play a more significant role in determining the overall performance. From the results, it can be seen that all the DL architectures with Swin-T achieved good effectiveness. The findings shown that using pre-trained CNN architectures for the categorization of pneumonia may provide exceptional levels of accuracy. Nevertheless, it is important to acknowledge that some algorithms, such as VGG19, had subpar performance, underscoring the need of choosing suitable architectures for a given job.

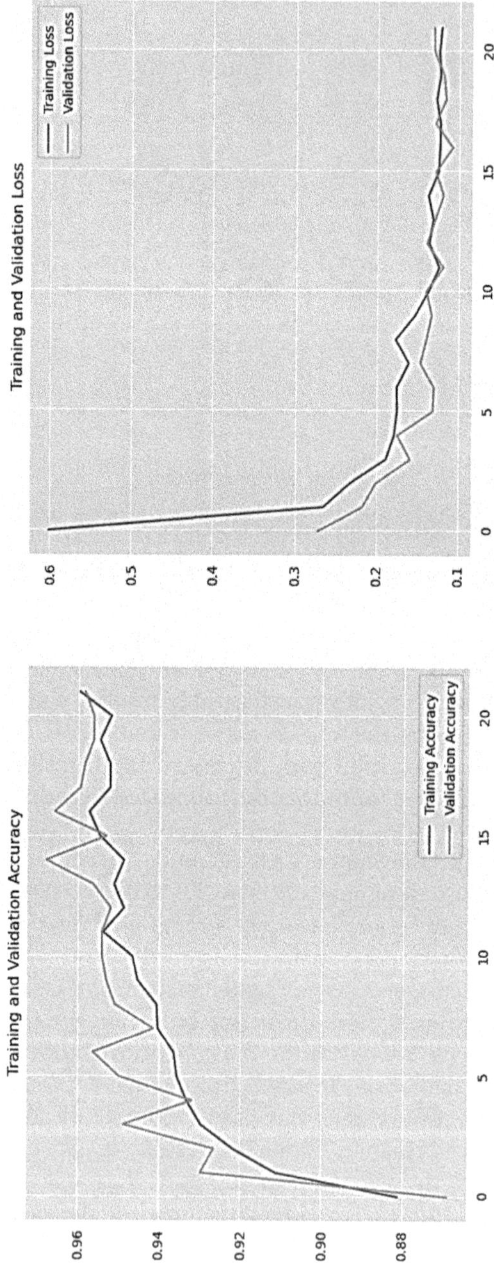

Figure 5.3 Accuracy and loss from EfficientNet-B0 + Swin-T configuration.

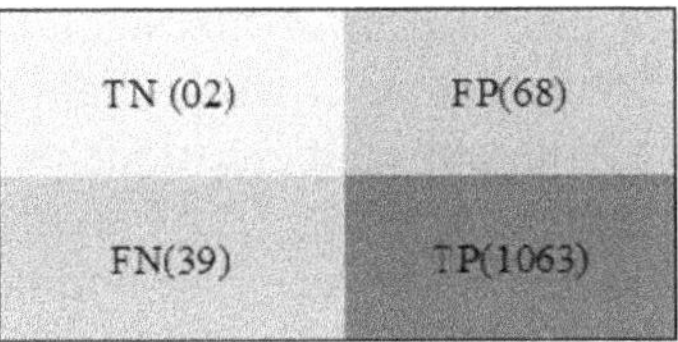

Figure 5.4 Confusion matrix for using extracted features from Swin-T and classification using EfficientNet-B0 CNN Architecture.

Utilizing ensemble learning with Swin-T has the potential to significantly enhance the efficacy of pneumonia detection. In addition, we examined the possible use of established DL models, such as ResNet-101, EfficientNet-B0, VGG16, and VGG19, for this specific purpose. The accuracy of Swin-T is an impressive 96.51%, showcasing its remarkable ability to accurately predict occurrences. The system's exceptional performance is validated by the Precision, Recall, and F1 Score metrics, which stand at 92.98%, 95.04%, and 94.01%, respectively.

As portrayed in Figure 5.3, the loss magnitude progressively diminished as the epoch count escalated from one to 25, further underscoring the model's refinement and convergence with extended training.

Figure 5.4 displays the confusion matrix for EfficientNet-B0 + Swin-T. The confusion matrix demonstrates the strong classification performance of the model, suggesting its effectiveness in reliably identifying both normal and positive class images.

5.5 CONCLUSION

The research provides valuable insights into the comparative performance of different DL architectures for diagnosing pneumonia using features extracted from Swin-T. The comprehensive investigation conducted in this study has successfully demonstrated the efficacy of combining various DL architectures, including ResNet-101, EfficientNet-B0, VGG16, and VGG19, with the Swin-T for the task of pneumonia diagnosis using the specified X-ray dataset. The results highlight the importance of selecting appropriate architectures and leveraging the complementary strengths of different DL approaches to achieve state-of-the-art performance. The EfficientNet-B0 + Swin-T model emerged as the top-performing configuration, achieving an impressive effectiveness. This underscores the synergistic relationship between the EfficientNet-B0 backbone and the Swin-T transformer, which enables effective capture of both local and global image features, leading to robust and accurate pneumonia classification. The ResNet-101 + Swin-T model also demonstrated strong performance, highlighting the value of the

ResNet-101 architecture's ability to extract hierarchical features, coupled with the attention-based mechanism of the Swin-T model. The VGG16 + Swin-T and VGG19 + Swin-T models, while slightly lower in performance compared to the other examined configurations, still achieved respectable results, showcasing the potential of the VGG architectures to benefit from integration with the Swin-T transformer. The findings of this study emphasize the critical role of model selection and architectural combination in designing effective DL-based image classification systems. By strategically leveraging the strengths of different DL models and the Swin-T transformer, practitioners can achieve state-of-the-art performance on a variety of image recognition tasks, including the diagnosis of pneumonia from chest X-ray images. Furthermore, future research could explore the use of other ensemble DL techniques to improve the classification accuracy.

REFERENCES

[1] G. Mackenzie, "The definition and classification of pneumonia," *Pneumonia*, vol. 8, no. 1, Aug. 2016, doi: 10.1186/s41479-016-0012-z

[2] "The top 10 causes of death," The top 10 causes of death, www.who.int/news-room/fact-sheets/detail/the-top-10-causes-of-death [Accessed: 21-Apr-2024].

[3] D. J. Alapat, M. V. Menon, and S. Ashok, "A review on detection of pneumonia in chest X-ray images using neural networks," *Journal of Biomedical Physics and Engineering*, vol. 12, no. 6, Dec. 2022, doi: 10.31661/jbpe.v0i0.2202-1461

[4] P. Mooney, "Chest X-ray images (pneumonia)," Kaggle, 24-Mar-2018. [Online]. Available: www.kaggle.com/datasets/paultimothymooney/chest-xray-pneumonia [Accessed: 22-Apr-2024].

[5] M. E. H. Chowdhury et al., "Can AI help in screening viral and COVID-19 pneumonia?" *IEEE Access*, vol. 8, pp. 132665–132676, 2020, doi: 10.1109/access.2020.3010287

[6] S. Kumar, and H. Kumar, "Lungcov: A diagnostic framework using machine learning and Imaging Modality," *International Journal on Technical and Physical Problems of Engineering (IJTPE)*, vol. 14, no. 51, Jun. 2022. http://mail.iotpe.com/IJTPE/IJTPE-2022/IJTPE-Issue51-Vol14-No2-Jun2022/23-IJTPE-Issue51-Vol14-No2-Jun2022-pp190-199.pdf

[7] D. Avola, A. Bacciu, L. Cinque, A. Fagioli, M. R. Marini, and R. Taiello, "Study on transfer learning capabilities for pneumonia classification in chest-x-rays images," *Computer Methods and Programs in Biomedicine*, vol. 221, p. 106833, Jun. 2022, doi: 10.1016/j.cmpb.2022.106833

[8] M. W. Kusk and S. Lysdahlgaard, "The effect of Gaussian noise on pneumonia detection on chest radiographs, using convolutional neural networks," *Radiography*, vol. 29, no. 1, pp. 38–43, Jan. 2023, doi: 10.1016/j.radi.2022.09.011

[9] Z. Liu et al., "Swin transformer: Hierarchical vision transformer using shifted windows," arXiv.org, Mar. 25, 2021. https://doi.org/10.48550/arXiv.2103.14030

[10] Y. Ma and W. Lv, "Identification of pneumonia in chest X-Ray image based on transformer," *International Journal of Antennas and Propagation*, vol. 2022, pp. 1–8, Aug. 2022, doi: 10.1155/2022/5072666.

[11] J. Jiang and S. Lin, "COVID-19 Detection in Chest X-ray Images Using Swin-Transformer and Transformer in Transformer," arXiv.org, Oct. 16, 2021. https://doi.org/10.48550/arXiv.2110.08427

[12] C. C. Ukwuoma et al., "A hybrid explainable ensemble transformer encoder for pneumonia identification from chest X-ray images," *Journal of Advanced Research*, vol. 48, pp. 191–211, Jun. 2023, doi: 10.1016/j.jare.2022.08.021.

[13] D. Li, "Attention-enhanced architecture for improved pneumonia detection in chest X-ray images," *BMC Medical Imaging*, vol. 24, no. 1, Jan. 2024, doi: 10.1186/s12880-023-01177-1.

[14] D. Kermany, K. Zhang, and M. H. Goldbaum, "Large Dataset of Labeled Optical Coherence Tomography (OCT) and Chest X-Ray Images," Jun. 01, 2018. http://data.mendeley.com/datasets/rscbjbr9sj/3

[15] "RSNA Pneumonia Detection Challenge | Kaggle." www.kaggle.com/competitions/rsna-pneumonia-detection-challenge/data

[16] R. Kundu, R. Das, Z. W. Geem, G.-T. Han, and R. Sarkar, "Pneumonia detection in chest X-ray images using an ensemble of deep learning models," *PLOS ONE*, vol. 16, no. 9, p. e0256630, Sep. 2021, doi: 10.1371/journal.pone.0256630.

[17] Z. Özdemır and H. Yalim Keleş, "Covid-19 Detection in Chest X-ray Images with Deep Learning," *2021 29th Signal Processing and Communications Applications Conference (SIU)*, IEEE, Jun. 2021, doi: 10.1109/siu53274.2021.9478028.

[18] G. Srivastava, N. Pradhan, and Y. Saini, "Ensemble of Deep Neural Networks based on Condorcet's Jury Theorem for screening Covid-19 and Pneumonia from radiograph images," *Computers in Biology and Medicine*, vol. 149, p. 105979, Oct. 2022, doi: 10.1016/j.compbiomed.2022.105979.

[19] A. Mabrouk, R. P. Díaz Redondo, A. Dahou, M. Abd Elaziz, and M. Kayed, "Pneumonia Detection on Chest X-ray Images Using Ensemble of Deep Convolutional Neural Networks," *Applied Sciences*, vol. 12, no. 13, p. 6448, Jun. 2022, doi: 10.3390/app12136448.

[20] T. Wang et al., "PneuNet: Deep learning for COVID-19 pneumonia diagnosis on chest X-ray image analysis using Vision Transformer," *Medical & Biological Engineering & Computing*, vol. 61, no. 6, pp. 1395–1408, Jan. 2023, doi: 10.1007/s11517-022-02746-2.

[21] S. Kumar and H. Kumar, "PneuML: A novel sequential convolutional neural network-based x-ray diagnostic system for pneumonia in contrast to machine learning and pre-trained networks," *U.P.B. Scientific Bulletin, Series C*, vol. 85, no. 4, pp. 119–136, 2023.

[22] S. Kumar and H. Kumar, "Classification of COVID-19 X-ray images using transfer learning with visual geometrical groups and novel sequential convolutional neural networks," *MethodsX*, vol. 11, p. 102295, Dec. 2023, doi: 10.1016/j.mex.2023.102295.

[23] M. E. H. Chowdhury et al., "Can AI Help in Screening Viral and COVID-19 Pneumonia?" *IEEE Access*, vol. 8, pp. 132665–132676, 2020, doi: 10.1109/access.2020.3010287.

[24] K. Simonyan and A. Zisserman, "Very deep convolutional networks for large-scale image recognition," arXiv preprint arXiv:1409.1556 preprint, 2014, 1–14.

[25] K. He, X. Zhang, S. Ren, and J. Sun, "Deep residual learning for image recognition," *Proceedings of the IEEE Conference on Computer Vision and Pattern Recognition (CVPR)*, IEEE, 2016, pp. 770–778, doi: 10.1109/CVPR.2016.90

[26] M. Tan and Q. Le, "EfficientNet: Rethinking Model Scaling for Convolutional Neural Networks," arXiv.org, May 28, 2019. https://doi.org/10.48550/arXiv.1905.11946

Chapter 6

The future of healthcare security
AI and cyber defenses

Ashutosh Bhatt and Ambika Aggarwal

6.1 INTRODUCTION

The healthcare industry is going through a radical change in the way medical services are administered and provided in a time of fast technology advancement. Modern technology is enabling this shift, and artificial intelligence (AI) is one of the main forces that could completely change the healthcare industry [1]. AI has the power to completely transform the healthcare industry by providing more precise diagnosis, individualized treatment regimens, and effective back-office operations [2].

Technology is a key factor in improving patient care, data management, and operational efficiency in the quickly changing field of healthcare [3]. But there are also previously unheard-of difficulties associated with this digital revolution, particularly in the area of cybersecurity. Healthcare companies are more vulnerable to cyberattacks as a result of their growing reliance on networked systems and storage of private patient data [4]. Advanced cyber defense mechanisms and artificial intelligence (AI) must work together to counter these threats. In exploring the future of healthcare security, this chapter focuses on the role that artificial intelligence (AI) and cyber defenses will play in protecting patient data and maintaining the integrity of healthcare networks. AI is adding value in many areas, but four areas remain the mainstay. Figure 6.1 shows four pillars of AI Applications in Healthcare these pillars are [2]:

1. Patient Care
2. Empowered Physician
3. Medical Imaging and Diagnostic
4. Research and Development

Technology breakthroughs have fueled a rapid evolution in the healthcare sector in recent years. Digital advancements, such as telemedicine and electronic health records (EHRs), have revolutionized the delivery of healthcare. But with all of this digital change, there are new difficulties as well, especially

DOI: 10.1201/9781003518075-6

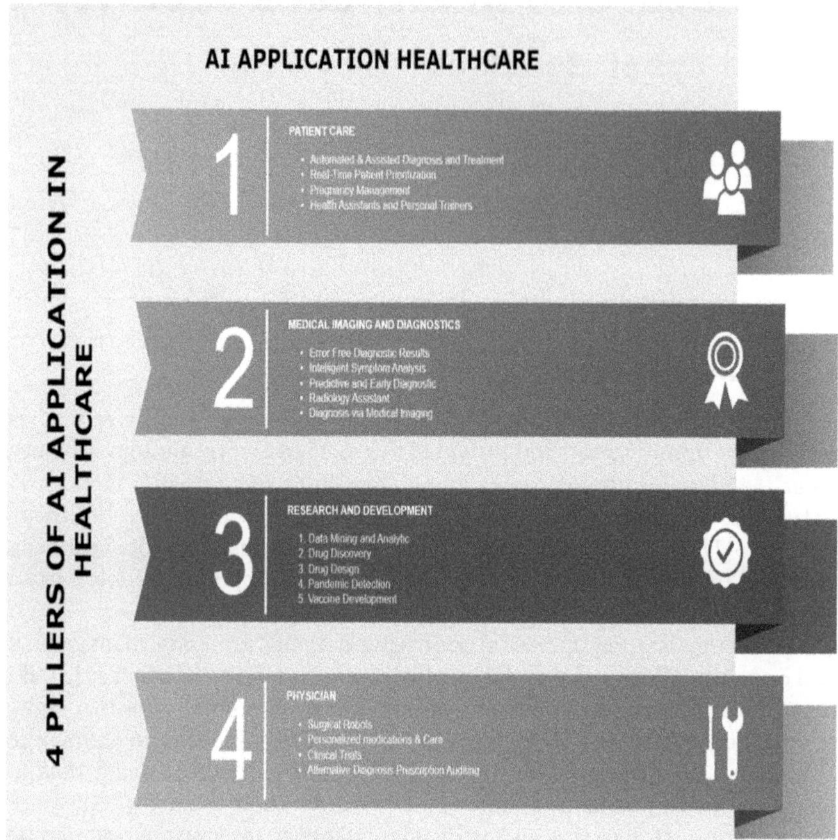

Figure 6.1 AI Applications in Healthcare.

with cybersecurity. Cybercriminals are increasingly focusing on healthcare institutions with ransomware attacks, data breaches, and phishing schemes among their targets [5].

Artificial intelligence (AI) and other cutting-edge technologies are being used by healthcare professionals to counter these risks and guarantee the security of patient information. This chapter examines the prospects and difficulties that lie ahead for the future of healthcare in the context of cybersecurity and artificial intelligence.

AI has a lot of potential for the healthcare industry because of its capacity to replicate human cognitive processes and carry out operations that previously required human intelligence. AI capabilities such as machine learning, computer vision, and natural language processing allow healthcare systems to quickly and efficiently analyze enormous

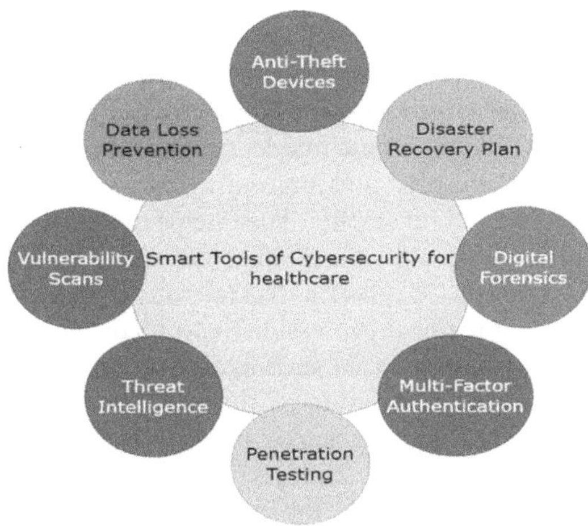

Figure 6.2 Tools of Cybersecurity for Healthcare.

information, identify intricate patterns, and provide actionable insights. Healthcare providers can improve clinical decision-making, optimize treatment plans, and more efficiently allocate resources by utilizing these capabilities. This will ultimately improve patient outcomes and streamline the healthcare system [6].

However, there are difficulties with integrating AI into healthcare, especially when it comes to protecting sensitive medical data. The potential of cyberattacks, data breaches, and other criminal acts rises as healthcare systems become increasingly electronically connected and dependent. Thus, protecting the security and privacy of patient information requires the confluence of AI and cybersecurity. To keep patients confident in healthcare systems, cyber threat prevention strategies need to be well thought out and put into action.

This study investigates the intricate connection between cybersecurity and AI in healthcare. With a focus on cybersecurity issues, AI's influence on healthcare procedures, and the rapidly changing technological landscape, this study seeks to offer a thorough knowledge of the ways in which these areas interact. This research aims to contribute to the creation of a safe and robust healthcare framework in Figure 6.2 that protects patient data and upholds trust by identifying vulnerabilities and offering practical ways for managing cyber hazards [7]. The convergence of artificial intelligence and cybersecurity in the field of healthcare represents a pivotal point in the history of healthcare innovation and patient-centered care, particularly at an era of unparalleled technical growth.

6.2 THE IMPACT OF AI AND CYBERSECURITY ON HEALTHCARE

AI has the potential to completely transform healthcare by lowering costs, enhancing operational effectiveness, and improving patient outcomes. AI-driven technologies, such as, machine learning and natural language processing, may examine massive information to find trends and insights that human specialists would miss [4]. This helps medical professionals to forecast the course of diseases, personalize treatment regimens, and make more accurate diagnoses. AI plays a crucial role in streamlining administrative tasks, allowing medical professionals to focus more on patient care. It achieves this by managing tasks such as insurance claim processing and appointment scheduling, thus reducing the workload on staff. Figure 6.3 depicts that AI in healthcare market is predicted to reach a valuation of around USD 187.95 billion by 2030, with a compound annual growth rate (CAGR) of 37%. In 2022, the market was valued at USD 15.1 billion. In 2022, the value of the North American AI healthcare sector was approximated at USD 6.8 billion [3].

The integration of AI and cybersecurity is transforming the healthcare sector, offering significant benefits and introducing new challenges. Here's an overview of their impact:

- **Better Patient Care:** Predictive analytics, customized treatment regimens, and more precise diagnosis are made possible by

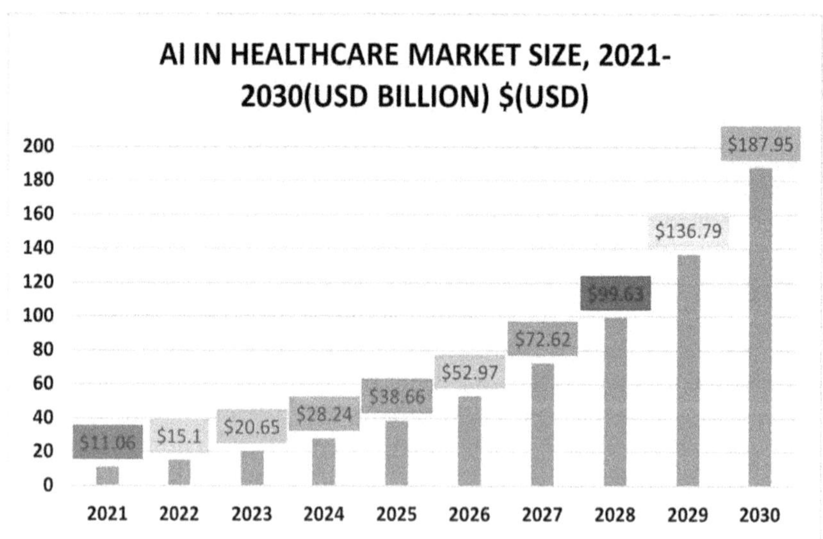

Figure 6.3 Healthcare Market Size. (Towards Healthcare.)

AI-powered solutions. Machine learning algorithms can analyze extensive patient data, uncovering patterns and trends that empower healthcare professionals to improve decision-making and enhance patient outcomes [8].

- **Enhanced Operational Efficiency:** Artificial Intelligence (AI) simplifies administrative duties like appointment scheduling, data processing for medical records, and inventory management. This increases productivity and frees up medical staff members to concentrate more on patient care [9].
- **Telemedicine and Remote Monitoring:** AI makes it possible for telemedicine systems and remote patient monitoring equipment to deliver on-demand healthcare services in real time. Patients who live in remote places or have mobility problems would particularly benefit from this as it eliminates the need for them to physically go in order to receive healthcare [10].
- **Cybersecurity Challenges:** Cybersecurity is an issue with the growing usage of AI and digital technology in healthcare. Because they handle sensitive data, healthcare businesses are often the target of cyberattacks. Healthcare services may be disrupted and patient data compromised by ransomware attacks, data breaches, and other cyber threats [11].
- **Data Privacy and Security:** In the medical field, patient data security is critical. AI can improve cybersecurity by immediately identifying and addressing threats. To protect patient information, access control, authentication, and encryption are crucial [12-13].
- **Regulatory Compliance:** To protect patient privacy and security, healthcare businesses must abide by laws like the Health Insurance Portability and Accountability Act (HIPAA). AI can assist in automating tasks related to compliance and guarantee that regulations are followed [14].

6.3 EXTENT AND FINANCIAL IMPACT OF GLOBAL CYBERATTACKS

The extent and financial impact of global cyberattacks vary widely depending on the nature and scale of the attack. However, some recent high-profile attacks provide a glimpse into the potential impact:

- **Ransomware Attacks:** Ransomware attacks are on the rise and can carry substantial financial consequences. For instance, the WannaCry ransomware attack of 2017, which impacted over 200,000 computers across 150 nations, resulting in an estimated $4 billion in damages [15].

- **Data Breaches:** Financial losses can stem from data breaches, incurred through expenses related to investigating the breach, notifying affected parties, and implementing security protocols to forestall future breaches. The financial impact can also include legal fees, regulatory fines, and reputational damage. For instance, the 2017 Equifax data breach impacted around 147 million individuals and led to a settlement exceeding $575 million [16, 17].
- **Business Email Compromise (BEC):** BEC attacks involve cybercriminals impersonating a company executive to trick employees into transferring money or sensitive information. Such attacks can cause substantial financial harm to organizations. For instance, in 2019, the FBI's Internet Crime Complaint Center (IC3) reported that BEC attacks led to losses exceeding $1.7 billion [18, 19].
- **Intellectual Property Theft:** Cyberattacks targeting the theft of intellectual property can inflict enduring financial repercussions on corporations. The theft of valuable intellectual property, such as trade secrets or proprietary technology, can result in lost revenue, competitive disadvantage, and damage to a company's reputation [20].

6.4 CYBERATTACKS: PHISHING, RANSOMWARE AND DATA BREACH TATISTICS: [21]

- 50% rise in cyberattacks over the previous year
- There will be 50% more weekly attacks in 2021 than in 2020.
- In 2021, the mean overall expense of a data breach climbed from $3.86 million to $4.24 million.
- Phishing assaults increased by 400% year over year in 2016.
- Data breaches requiring longer response times (exceeding 200 days) incur an average cost of $4.87 million, whereas breaches necessitating shorter reaction times (under 200 days) average at $3.61 million.
- Networks with an estimated vulnerability of 93% to cyberattacks
- Estimated cybersecurity spending by 2025 is $458.9 billion.

Global cyberattacks have a large financial impact overall, and this cost will only increase as cybercriminals get more skilled and assaults happen more frequently. Businesses need to make significant investments in cybersecurity defenses in order to fend off these attacks and reduce the financial risks involved. In recent years, the healthcare business has been a primary target for cyberattacks and has seen several difficulties, especially in the provider sector. Numerous businesses rely on antiquated and unsafe legacy IT systems, which leaves them open to online attacks [15]. With more devices connected, there is a greater attack surface and greater difficulty in securing them due to the rise of the Internet of Medical Things (IoMT). As a result,

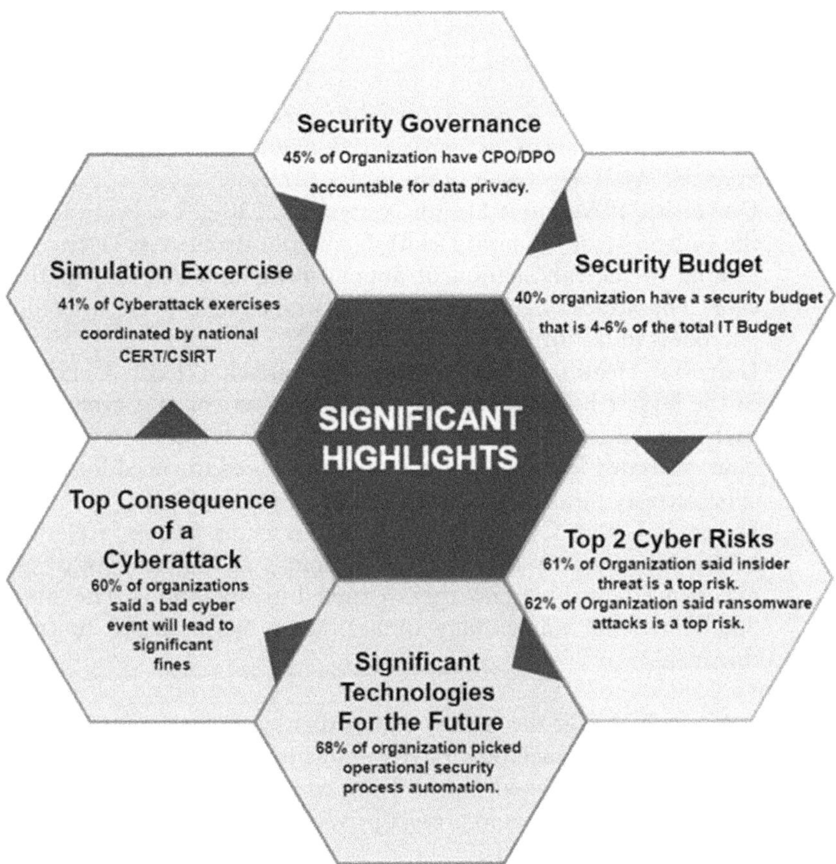

Figure 6.4 Cybersecurity Trends in the Healthcare Sector.

cybersecurity threats are increasingly directly threatening patient safety rather than just data breaches [11].

Cybersecurity 2019 research, Wipro polled 211 firms in six industries and 27 countries to gain a comprehensive landscape (Figure 6.4) of the global cybersecurity.

Several high-profile cyberattacks have targeted the healthcare industry in recent years, highlighting the vulnerability of medical systems and the importance of cybersecurity in healthcare. Here are some notable examples:

- **WannaCry Ransomware Attack (2017):** WannaCry, one of the most pervasive cyberattacks in history, compromised over 200,000 machines across 150 nations, including medical facilities. Due to the ransomware attack, hospitals and clinics in the UK were forced to cancel appointments and redirect patients, which had a significant negative impact on the National Health Service (NHS) [22].

- **NotPetya Cyberattack (2017):** Initially disguising itself as a software update, NotPetya was a ransomware attack that affected companies all around the world, including medical facilities. Numerous healthcare organizations experienced operational disruptions and financial losses as a result of the attack [22].
- **University of Vermont Health Network (2020):** A cyberattack on the University of Vermont Health Network disrupted its IT systems, leading to the cancellation of appointments and delays in patient care. The attack highlighted the importance of cybersecurity preparedness in healthcare organizations [22].
- **Universal Health Services (UHS) Cyberattack (2020):** UHS, one of the largest hospital chains in the US, experienced a cyberattack that affected its IT systems and forced some facilities to resort to manual record-keeping. The attack underscored the need for robust cybersecurity measures in the healthcare sector [22].
- **Fresenius Group Cyberattack (2020):** Fresenius Group, a German healthcare company that operates hospitals and clinics worldwide, experienced a cyberattack that disrupted its operations. The attack highlighted the vulnerability of healthcare organizations to cyber threats [22].

These instances highlight the serious effects that cyberattacks can have on the healthcare industry, including interruptions to patient treatment, monetary losses, and reputational harm. They emphasize the importance of robust cybersecurity measures to protect private patient data and ensure the reliability of healthcare systems.

6.5 CYBERSECURITY CONUNDRUM IN HEALTHCARE

The necessity to weigh the advantages of digital innovation against the dangers of cyberattacks characterizes the cybersecurity conundrum that the healthcare sector faces. Digital innovations including electronic health records (EHRs), connected medical equipment, and telemedicine hold promise for bettering patient care, increasing operational effectiveness, and providing remote access to healthcare. However, these technologies also bring with them new weaknesses that hackers might take advantage of. Because healthcare businesses store important data, such as confidential patient information and intellectual property, they are often the targets of cyberattacks [23].

The healthcare cybersecurity dilemma is exacerbated by several factors:

- **Growing Complexity:** Thanks to linked networks, a plethora of digital tools, and applications, healthcare systems are getting more and more complicated. It is difficult to guarantee the system's overall security because of its complexity [23].

- **Lack of Resources:** A lot of healthcare businesses don't have the funding or the qualified staff necessary to handle cybersecurity issues. They may become open to cyberattacks as a result [23].
- **Regularity Requirements:** Strict legislative standards, such as those outlined in the United States' 'Health Insurance Portability and Accountability Act (HIPAA)', govern how well healthcare firms protect patient information. There may be heavy fines and reputational harm for noncompliance [23].
- **Human Factors:** Whether via phishing attempts, careless handling of private data, or insufficient employee training, human error continues to play a big role in cybersecurity breaches. [23]

Healthcare businesses need to have a holistic strategy to cybersecurity that encompasses the following in order to handle the cybersecurity challenge in healthcare [22]:

- Putting strong cybersecurity safeguards in place, like frequent security audits, access controls, and encryption.
- Putting money into staff cybersecurity awareness and training programs will lower the possibility of human error.
- Exchanging threat intelligence and best practices with government organizations and business partners.
- Ensuring adherence to industry norms and legal obligations for data protection.

By addressing these challenges and implementing effective cybersecurity measures, healthcare organizations can mitigate the risks posed by cyber threats and protect the integrity of their systems and the confidentiality of patient information.

6.6 ADVANCING AI IN CYBERSECURITY: A PATH FORWARD

The future of AI and cybersecurity holds great promise, but it also presents several challenges that must be addressed. Here are some key considerations for moving forward:

- **Improved AI-driven Cyber Defense:** AI can be used to create more sophisticated cybersecurity defenses. AI-powered solutions help enterprises stay ahead of hostile actors by detecting and responding to cyber threats instantly. AI technologies will become more and more significant in cybersecurity as they develop. [18]

- **Enhanced Threat Intelligence:** Artificial intelligence (AI) can enhance threat intelligence by sifting through enormous volumes of data to find patterns and trends that point to potential cyberthreats. Organizations can gain a better understanding of and ability to minimize cyber threats by utilizing AI for threat intelligence. [19]
- **Prioritize Privacy and Ethics:** As AI becomes more widely used in cybersecurity, privacy and ethics must come first. AI systems need to be developed and put into use in a way that respects user privacy and adheres to all applicable laws and guidelines. [18]
- **Cooperation and Information Sharing:** Organizations, governments, and business partners must work together to combat cybersecurity, which is a team effort. Through the exchange of threat intelligence and best practices, all parties involved can enhance their cybersecurity posture [18].
- **Investment in Cybersecurity Abilities:** As the need for cybersecurity experts increases, so does the amount of money allocated to the development of cybersecurity abilities. Businesses should spend money on educating and enhancing the skills of their employees in order to handle the changing cybersecurity environment [17].
- **Constant System Monitoring and Adaptation:** Because cyber threats are always changing, businesses need to keep an eye on their systems and modify their cybersecurity plans as necessary. AI can assist in automating this process by instantly recognizing and neutralizing new threats [18].
- **Regulatory Compliance:** Organizations must adhere to cybersecurity laws, rules, and guidelines. Organizations can reduce their risk of regulatory fines and reputational harm by maintaining compliance [18].
- **Cybersecurity Awareness:** Lastly, it's critical that staff members and end users understand cybersecurity. Employers should teach their staff the value of upholding a robust security posture and cybersecurity best practices [16].

6.7 STRATEGIES FOR STRENGTHENING CYBERSECURITY MEASURES

Businesses need cybersecurity to stay in operation, especially in industries like healthcare where patient care and safety are at risk. A healthcare organization's digital infrastructure can be compromised, which can have dire repercussions [14]. Taking action to guarantee that the digital environment is safe and secure for use is essential. All levels should be subject to these safeguards, which should begin at the entrance point (such as the firewall) and work their way down to safeguarding end users' computers by preventing access and banning USB connections.

- Starting at the top, or the end user level, are the first steps in this direction. Any type of application or data should only be accessed by means of a well specified approval matrix that is thoroughly documented [9]. The basis for all access control should be roles. Without adhering to the correct permission hierarchy, no access should be granted.
- All approved applications must implement multifactor authentication for login.
- Internet connectivity and USB ports should be disabled unless absolutely essential. If these actions are necessary, they must be executed safely within a separate network to safeguard the primary network's integrity.
- The use of pen drives has decreased dramatically in recent years due to the widespread availability of online storage solutions like Google Drive and Microsoft OneDrive. With the help of these online drives, users may store their data in a cloud with already-installed robust security and access it from any location, doing away with the need for physical devices to exchange the data. Users can exchange information from these online drives to anybody, anywhere in the globe, from any device (desktop, laptop, or smartphone). In every healthcare institution, the most vital and significant type of information is patient data, which is kept on servers and data storage devices. It is crucial to guarantee the availability and security of this data. It is imperative that this data remain accessible around-the-clock all year long.
- Encrypted formats should be used to hold patient data, regardless of whether it is kept in a database, medical picture, or scanned paper [24]. This guarantees that the data cannot be read or altered even in the event that an outside party obtains access to it.
- This data should be kept in two separate locations to improve security and availability even more. Retaining a live copy of the production data at a different location is essential for Business Continuity Planning (BCP) and Disaster Recovery(DR) [20].
- For example, the organization's operations that depend on this data would stop if an outside party was able to get past the firewalls, access the data, and encrypt it. Nonetheless, the company can easily carry on if a real-time replica of this data is accessible at another secure location.

6.8 OTHER ESSENTIAL STRATEGIES FOR SHAPING THE FUTURE OF HEALTHCARE

- **Embracing Technology:** Utilizing digital tools to improve patient care, increase efficiency, and facilitate remote monitoring, such as wearable technology, telemedicine, and health applications.

- **Data Analytics and AI:** Utilizing big data and artificial intelligence (AI) to extract insights, forecast patterns, customize therapies, and maximize resource allocation is known as data analytics.
- **Focus on Prevention and Population Health:** Prioritizing population health management and wellness while abandoning a treatment-focused, reactive approach in favor of a proactive, preventive one.
- **Interdisciplinary Collaboration:** In order to spur innovation and enhance the provision of healthcare, interdisciplinary collaboration is encouraged by researchers, policymakers, healthcare practitioners, and technology specialists.
- **Patient-Centered Care:** Patient-centered care involves putting the needs, preferences, and results of each individual patient front and center and incorporating them in the decision-making process.
- **Value-Based Care:** Changing the way healthcare is delivered by rewarding providers according to patient outcomes and overall quality of care rather than quantity of services rendered.
- **Addressing Social Determinants of Health:** Recognizing and treating the influence of environmental, social, and economic factors on health outcomes is necessary to achieve health equity. This is known as addressing social determinants of health [23].
- **Education and Training:** To stay up to date with new treatments, technology, and best practices, healthcare workers should invest in ongoing education and training.
- **Regulatory adaptation:** Regulatory adaptation is the process of modifying legal frameworks to take into account new developments, encourage creativity, and protect patient privacy and safety.
- **Global Cooperation:** Promoting worldwide cooperation to exchange resources, research results, and best practices in order to address global health issues.

Implementing ethical guidelines and governance frameworks in AI/Cybersecurity development and deployment: Table 6.1 discusses various guidelines for AI and cybersecurity to be implemented in the healthcare field.

6.9 CONTINUOUS MONITORING AND UPDATES

Although the aforementioned methods encompass a substantial aspect of cybersecurity, it is imperative to tackle even the smallest vulnerabilities that may jeopardize security. It is crucial to continuously monitor each step of the cycle, from data gathering to deployment.

To find any compromise, routine system health checks should be carried out. To keep cybersecurity secure, periodic vulnerability assessments and penetration tests, or VAPTs, are essential. User Acceptance Testing (UAT) and deployment environments should be included in these tests as well as

Table 6.1 Ethical Guidelines for AI and Cybersecurity

S.N	*Ethical Guideline For AI*	*Ethical Guideline For Cybersecurity*
1.	Define a set of ethical principles that should guide AI development and deployment in your organization. These principles should cover concerns related to transparency, fairness, accountability, and privacy.	Define a set of ethical principles that should guide cybersecurity development and deployment. These principles should tackle concerns such as transparency, privacy, accountability, and respect for human rights.
2.	Establish a governance framework to oversee AI development and deployment. This framework should include processes for risk assessment, decision-making, and monitoring the impact of AI systems	Establish a governance framework to oversee cybersecurity development and deployment. This framework should include processes for risk assessment, decision-making, and monitoring the impact of cybersecurity measures.
3.	Educate employees, partners, and other stakeholders about the ethical guidelines and governance framework. Ensure that everyone involved in AI development and deployment understands their roles and responsibilities.	Educate employees, partners, and other stakeholders about the ethical guidelines and governance framework. Ensure that everyone involved in cybersecurity understands their roles and responsibilities.
4.	Integrate ethical considerations into every stage of the AI development lifecycle, from design to deployment. This includes identifying potential biases in training data, ensuring transparency in decision-making algorithms, and providing mechanisms for redress if AI systems cause harm.	Integrate ethical considerations into every stage of the cybersecurity development lifecycle, from planning to implementation. This includes considering the potential impact of cybersecurity measures on individuals and society.
5.	Continuously monitor and evaluate the impact of AI systems on individuals and society. Use this information to update your ethical guidelines and governance framework as needed.	Continuously monitor and evaluate the effectiveness of cybersecurity measures. Use this information to update your ethical guidelines and governance framework as needed.
6.	Engage with external stakeholders, such as regulators, civil society organizations, and affected communities, to ensure that your ethical guidelines and governance framework are robust and effective.	Engage with external stakeholders, such as regulators, industry groups, and affected communities, to ensure that your ethical guidelines and governance framework are robust and effective.
7.	Be transparent about your AI systems and their capabilities. Provide clear explanations of how decisions are made and give users the option to opt out of using AI-driven services if they are uncomfortable with them.	Be transparent about your cybersecurity measures and their capabilities. Provide clear explanations of how cybersecurity decisions are made and how they affect individuals and society.
8.	Continuously iterate and improve your ethical guidelines and governance framework based on feedback and lessons learned from AI development and deployment.	Collaborate with other organizations and share best practices for ethical cybersecurity development and deployment. This can help raise standards across the industry.

production settings. VAPT assists in locating current vulnerabilities and possible hazards. It is critical to warn about these hazards in a timely manner.

Raising awareness of these hazards throughout the entire project team can aid in the root-cause management of many problems. The techniques outlined above can be used to manage any residual hazards. It's critical to remember that threats related to technology, particularly artificial intelligence (AI) and other technologies, are always changing. As such, our strategies for reducing cyber threats need to change as well. To keep abreast of new risks, we need to constantly enhance our systems, instruments, and procedures.

6.10 AI AS A KEY COMPONENT IN ENHANCING CYBERSECURITY

AI plays a significant role in strengthening cybersecurity by enhancing threat detection, response capabilities, and overall system resilience. Here's how AI contributes to cybersecurity:

- **Threat detection:**
  AI systems are able to examine enormous volumes of data and identify trends that could point to possible security vulnerabilities. Anomalies in user behavior, system configurations, and network traffic that could indicate a cyberattack can be recognized using machine learning models.
- **Real-time Monitoring:**
  AI-powered solutions have the ability to continuously watch over networks and systems in real time, sending out alerts right away if anything seems fishy. By taking a proactive stance, organizations may react quickly to possible dangers.
- **Behavioral Analysis:**
  AI may examine user behavior to spot patterns that deviate from the norm, which can be used to find compromised accounts or insider threats.
- **Automated Response:**
  Artificial Intelligence (AI) can reduce response times and mitigate the effects of attacks by automating actions in response to specific cyberthreats. Examples of these actions include isolating compromised computers or blocking suspicious IP addresses.
- **Vulnerability Management:**
  AI can help find and rank software and system vulnerabilities so that companies can fix important problems before hackers take advantage of them.

- **Phishing Detection:**
  To help users avoid falling for fraudulent schemes, artificial intelligence (AI) systems can examine emails and other communication channels to identify phishing attempts.
- **Enhanced Authentication:**
  By examining user activity patterns, Artificial Intelligence (AI) may enhance authentication procedures and make them more safe and smooth.
- **Adaptive security:**
  Adaptive security refers to AI's ability to adjust its algorithms and models in response to fresh data, allowing it to keep up with emerging cyberthreats.

6.11 CONCLUSION

The intersection of AI and cybersecurity presents a significant opportunity in the field of healthcare technology development. AI is creating new opportunities for medical advancement, but it also presents cybersecurity issues that need to be handled carefully. At this critical juncture, emerging leaders are in the vanguard and are entrusted with driving innovation while protecting patient data and system resilience. These future leaders in healthcare have a variety of duties. By informing and bringing attention to the intricacies of cybersecurity and AI, they need to establish their path is steered by moral precepts, promoting AI-powered solutions reinforced by cybersecurity protocols. They support a well-balanced regulatory structure that fosters innovation and protects patient interests. These future leaders must lead proactive defense in addressing issues like resource constraints, human error, networked systems, and compliance. These leaders' commitment to ethical behavior, constant adaptability, and cooperative approaches will help to create a healthcare environment that embraces AI's promise while maintaining patient trust as technology continues on its disruptive journey. Their inspiring leadership guides us toward a safe, cutting-edge, and patient-centered healthcare future amidst this dynamic convergence.

REFERENCES

1. J. D. Smith, "Artificial intelligence in healthcare: Anticipating challenges to ethics," *AMA Journal of Ethics*, vol. 21, no. 2, pp. E167–E173, 2019.
2. E. J. Topol, "High-performance medicine: The convergence of human and artificial intelligence," *Nature Medicine*, vol. 25, no. 1, pp. 44–56, Jan. 2019.
3. A. Esteva et al., "Dermatologist-level classification of skin cancer with deep neural networks," *Nature*, vol. 542, no. 7639, pp. 115–118, 2017.

4.   A. Rajkomar, J. Dean, and I. Kohane, "Machine learning in medicine," *New England Journal of Medicine*, vol. 380, no. 14, pp. 1347–1358, 2019.

5.   N. Kshetri, "Cybersecurity in healthcare: A systematic review of modern threats and trends," *Technology in Society*, vol. 49, pp. 65–76, 2017.

6.   N. M. Patel, J. Schirm, and S. Lakhani, "Safeguarding the digital hospital: Cybersecurity in the age of rapid technological advancement," *American Journal of Roentgenology*, vol. 214, no. 6, pp. 1235–1241, 2020.

7.   B. Lee, A. M. Kuo, and I. S. Kohane, "Transparent machine learning models for predicting diagnosis codes in electronic health records," *Journal of the American Medical Informatics Association*, vol. 25, no. 7, pp. 887–893, 2018.

8.   D. S. Char et al., "Deep learning and the future of electronic health records," *NPJ Digital Medicine*, vol. 1, no. 1, pp. 1–6, 2018.

9.   S. M. McKinney et al., "International evaluation of an AI system for breast cancer screening," *Nature*, vol. 577, no. 7788, pp. 89–94, 2020.

10.   Z. Obermeyer and E. J. Emanuel, "Predicting the future – Big data, machine learning, and clinical medicine," *New England Journal of Medicine*, vol. 375, no. 13, pp. 1216–1219, 2016.

11.   J. H. Chen and S. M. Asch, "Machine Learning and Prediction in Medicine — Beyond the Peak of Inflated Expectations," *The New England Journal of Medicine*, vol. 376, no. 26, pp. 2507–2509, 2017.

12.   C. Rajat, P. Singh, and A. Agarwal, "A security solution for the transmission of confidential data and efficient file authentication based on DES, AES, DSS and RSA." *International Journal of Innovative Technology and Exploring Engineering*, vol. 1, no. 3, p. 5, 2012.

13.   T. Jadczyk et al., "Artificial intelligence can improve patient management at the time of a pandemic: the role of voice technology," *Journal Medical Internet Research*, vol. 23, no. 5, pp. e22959, May 2021.

14.   V. Božić, "Use of artificial intelligence in healthcare," 2023. [Online]. Available: 10.13140/RG.2.2.35096.88322.

15.   C. Hale, "Impact of Artificial Intelligence on Healthcare Cybersecurity," www.linkedin.com. [Online]. Available: www.linkedin.com/pulse/impact-artificial-intelligence-healthcare-charles-hale/.

16.   M. Ahola, "The Role of Human Error in Successful Cyber Security Breaches," 2022. [Online]. Available: https://blog.usecure.io/the-role-of-human-error-in-successful-cyber-security-breaches.

17.   A. Agarwal, N. Bora, and N. Arora, "Goodput enhanced digital image watermarking scheme based on DWT and SVD," *International Journal of Application or Innovation in Engineering & Management*, vol. 2, no. 9, pp. 36–41, 2013.

18.   G. Slabodkin, "Insulin pumps among millions of devices facing risk from newly disclosed cyber vulnerability, IBM says," MedTech Dive, Aug. 25, 2020. [Online]. Available: www.medtechdive.com/news/insulin-pumps-among-millions-of-iot-devices-vulnerable-to-hacker-attacks/584043/.

19.   "Anthem medical data breach," May 27, 2023. [Online]. Available: https://en.wikipedia.org/wiki/Anthem_medical_data_breach.

20. P. Kumar, R. Chaudhary, A. Aggarwal, P. Singh, and R. Tomar, "Improving medical image segmentation techniques using multiphase level set approach via bias correction," *International Journal of Engineering and Advanced Technology*, vol. 1, no. 5, Jun 2012.

21. S. C. Apps, "Cyberattacks 2021: Statistics From the Last Year | Spanning," *Spanning*, Feb. 9, 2023. [Online]. Available: https://spanning.com/blog/cyberattacks-2021-phishing-ransomware-data-breach-statistics/#:~:text=According%20to%20Check%20Point%20Research,in%202021%20compared%20to%202020.

22. "Cyber attacks on Indian healthcare industry second highest in the world: CloudSEK," *The Hindu*, Sep. 20, 2022. [Online]. Available: www.thehindu.com/sci-tech/technology/cyber-attacks-on-indian-healthcare-industry-second-highest-in-the-world-cloudsek/article65914129.ece#:~:text=%22India%20recorded%20the%20second%20highest,records%2C%20according%20to%20the%20report.

23. K. Preeti, A. Singh, and A. Bhatt, "Detection Techniques Used For Foodborne Pathogens and Its Significant Financial and Human Behavioral Effects," *Journal for ReAttach Therapy and Developmental Diversities*, vol. 6, no. 2s, pp. 181–184, 2023.

24. "5 AIIMS Servers Hacked, 1.3 TB Data Encrypted in Recent Cyberattack, Govt Tells RS," *The Wire*. [Online]. Available: https://thewire.in/government/aiims-servers-cyberattack-ransomware-rajya-sabha.

Chapter 7

An efficient machine learning approach to mitigate DDoS attacks in Ad-hoc networks

*Rashid Rafiq Shah, Honey Sharma,
Amandeep Singh Kalra, and Nipun Sharma*

7.1 INTRODUCTION

A sensor network is like a pop-up team that forms quickly for a specific job. It's a big area of study, and people often have meetings about it. A Sensor Network is like a team of tiny sensors (like minicomputers) that can sense things, talk to each other without wires, and do some thinking. There can be a lot of them, hundreds or even thousands. Sometimes, these sensors have trouble talking to each other, which can slow things down and use up more energy. People are working on ways to make this better by making it more secure and using less energy.

Depending on how the sensors are organized, they can be like a group where everyone has the same job, or they can be organized into smaller groups with one leader in each group (Sidhu & Sachdeva, 2020).

One way to save energy is by organizing the sensors into groups (clusters) and having a leader in each group. This leader helps pass along information.

Sensor Networks are groups of little sensors spread out in different places. They keep an eye on things like temperature, sound, and pressure. Making sure they're secure is important, especially in real-world situations. Making sure the sensors use their energy wisely is a big challenge. There are different ways to help them find the best routes for sending information, which can help them last longer.

In this approach, we will be looking at how to use a mix of two methods to use less energy. We'll be using a computer program called MATLAB to pretend and see how it would work. We will do a bunch of pretend tests to see which method is the best for saving energy and making everything run smoothly, including network performance like energy consumption (Joules), packet delivery ratio, throughput (Mbps). A sensor network is like a group of sites that can talk to each other without needing a central system to control them. They're like a bunch of friends who can chat directly, even when they're moving around. But, because they don't have a boss overseeing everything, they can be more vulnerable to problems. Imagine a group of friends playing a game without a referee—sometimes things can get tricky!

DOI: 10.1201/9781003518075-7

Security is a big concern for Ad-hoc-Network (MANET). They need to make sure their conversations are private and safe from any sneaky intruders. Just like making sure no one eavesdrops on your private talks. There are different types of attacks that can happen in Ad-hoc-Network, like tricks that try to disrupt the communication. It's important to be aware of these potential issues and have ways to protect against them.

In this study, they're going to figure out how to save energy in an Ad-hoc-Network by using a special method called OLSR. It's like finding a smarter way for these devices to talk to each other while using less energy. A network is like a group of three or more computers that work together, sort of like a team. They share information with each other, kind of like passing notes in class. Wi-Fi is a cool technology that lets computers talk to each other without needing wires. It's like magic radio waves that let them communicate.

7.2 PROBLEM STATEMENT

Sensor networks are comprised of autonomous sensor nodes that are spread in space to monitor various physical or environmental factors, including but not limited to temperature, sound, and pressure, at diverse geographical locations. Sensor networks are susceptible to a multitude of uncertainties. The primary uncertainties in ad hoc networks pertain to the Physical, MAC, and network layers, which play crucial roles in the routing mechanism. Attacks targeting the network layer often serve two primary objectives: obstructing the transmission of packets or manipulating routing messages by introducing modifications to certain parameters. One example of a cyber assault is flooding, specifically in the context of a DDoS attack. Many different methods have been created for making communication work in ad hoc networks. It is not feasible for one solution to effectively mitigate all forms of assaults in Ad-hoc Networks. This study aims to propose an innovative approach to addressing the impact of uncertainty and improving network performance.

7.3 OBJECTIVES

The objectives are declared below:

1. To study the analysis of uncertainties in sensor networks and their pros and cons.
2. To implement the machine learning and optimize approach to mitigate the DDoS attack.
3. To evaluate how well the proposed approach works in terms of the legitimate traffic and DDoS traffic for high network lifetime.

7.4 LITERATURE SURVEY

Dhingra and Sachdeva (2021) proposed a method that employs a cascaded multi-classifier two-phase approach to detect and classify incoming traffic for potential intrusions. By breaking the process into two phases, it focuses on efficient detection while enabling specific categorization of threats like DDoS attacks or flash events. This strategy aims to balance accuracy and computational efficiency, crucial for real-time monitoring systems. Ultimately, it promises to enhance network security by swiftly identifying and responding to potential threats, covertly bolstering defenses.

Korir and Cheruiyot (2022) examined security challenges in mobile Ad-hoc Networks due to dynamic topology and node mobility. It reviews existing protocols, categorizing them as proactive or reactive, highlighting their merits and challenges. Ultimately, it calls for more efficient and secure routing protocols to optimize network performance, suggesting ideal features for future development.

Reddy and Thilagam (2020) proposed a solution that integrates network node authentication and a naïve Bayes classifier to effectively identify and isolate DDoS attack patterns, as demonstrated by superior performance in simulations. Ultimately, it aims to secure legitimate traffic from DDoS attacks.

Sidhu and Sachdeva (2020) proposed a solution that Wireless Sensor Networks (WSNs) are important because they can be used in many ways, like monitoring and collecting data. However, keeping these networks secure is a big challenge, especially since their routing protocols can be easily attacked. This approach particularly focused on routing protocols. It highlights the security problems in ZigBee Wireless Sensor Networks and the Ad-hoc On-Demand Distance Vector routing protocol.

Chuang, Liu, and Tsai (2022) proposed a solution for detection of abnormal attacks using an AI module integrated into the SDN topology. Machine learning algorithms such as decision trees, random forests, bagging, AdaBoost, and deep learning models are highlighted for their effectiveness in detecting DDoS attacks. The AI module not only identifies but also acts against the attack source, enhancing the overall flexibility and security of the network architecture.

Rasool, Ashraf, Ahmed, Wang, Rafique, and Anwar (2019) proposed a solution that detect flooding attacks. CyberPulse enhances the ability to detect and mitigate LFAs, ensuring more robust network security. The results indicate that CyberPulse uses traffic filtering methods, offering a practical solution to safeguard SDN environments from malicious activities.

Liu, Gu, and Wang (2021) proposed a solution with the development of an intrusion detection system (IDS) that aims to protect digital assets from network security threats. Traditional IDSs often struggle with timely alerts and accuracy. To address these issues, the paper proposes a new IDS model that combines machine learning and deep learning techniques.

Bawany, Shamsi, and Salah (2017) propose a new framework tailored for large-scale networks, such as smart cities built on SDN infrastructure. This framework aims to meet application-specific requirements for DDoS detection and mitigation, offering improved scalability, accuracy, and adaptability.

Zeng, Cheng, Cao, Yang, and Sheng (2023) propose a new method called the Adaptive Clustering-based LightGBM (AcLGB) for detecting DDoS attacks. This method introduces a lightweight approach to classify DDoS traffic effectively.

Harithaa and Vijayalakshmi (2023), proposed a solution called machine learning approach to detect and mitigate DDoS attack. Machine learning techniques can analyze large amounts of network traffic data, identify insights inside the data, and detect anomalies indicative of DDoS activity.

Behal, Kumar and Sachdeva (2018) Proposed a method that shows how to detect patterns from DDoS attack and legitimate traffic. D-FAC offers a novel solution by using the *I*-Divergence metric and distributing computational tasks to PoP routers, leading to better performance and efficiency in protecting against these attacks.

7.5 PROPOSED WORK

Sensor networks are collections of small, independent sensors placed in different locations to monitor things like temperature, sound, and pressure. One major challenge in these networks is energy consumption, especially since the nodes are battery powered. Quality of Service (QOS) optimization is crucial because of this energy constraint. Many protocols have been developed to minimize errors in routing, which is essential for prolonging the network's lifespan. The effectiveness of sensor networks largely depends on the routing protocol used. Research in mobile Ad-hoc Networks have focused on secure routing for long-distance information transmission. These networks operate without a fixed infrastructure and are employed for monitoring various systems. The field of sensor networks is dynamic, each year, many workshops and conferences are organized and conducted. A sensor network comprises hundreds or even thousands of tiny sensors capable of sensing, communicating wirelessly, and performing computational tasks. These networks find applications in diverse fields such as military, disaster management, healthcare, industry, and more, each with unique requirements. This chapter focuses on efficient protocols to optimize sensor networks. The previous work has emphasized energy conservation in security processes, but there's room for improvement in terms of energy efficiency (Chuang, Liu, and Tsai, 2022). The proposed approach employs both Moth Flame Optimization and Back Propagation Neural Network techniques. This method aims to reduce uncertainties and enhance packet deliveries and throughputs in the network.

7.6 IMPLEMENTATION

Figure 7.1 shows network creation in which nodes are deployed, the communication is done as per network nodes. The Nodes are plotted blue in color and show that the packet sending as per DDoS attack occurred during transmissions. The blue line shows the link among the nodes which are transmitting packets in the sensor networks (Behal, Kumar, and Sachdeva, 2018).

Figure 7.2 shows the request increases on the networks due to the DDoS effect. This then shows that the loading on the nodes increases to a certain limit where the congestion among the networks is great enough that overhead consumption and failures among the nodes occurs (Rasool, Ashraf, Ahmed, Wang, Rafique, and Anwar, 2019).

Figure 7.3 shows the training of the network and shows that the new method is good at providing effective training and getting good results in reducing the error rates in the performance of the system in a back propagation scenario (Chuang, Liu, & Tsai, 2022)

Figure 7.4 shows the DDoS traffic classifications in this machine learning approach demonstrates its capability to successfully classify traffic patterns. In terms of DDoS traffic it mitigates and regulates transmissions, which is a significant approach for the efficient network lifetime.

Figure 7.5 shows that the base station can distinguish between incoming traffic: DDoS traffic or legitimate traffic (Sidhu & Sachdeva, 2020). The

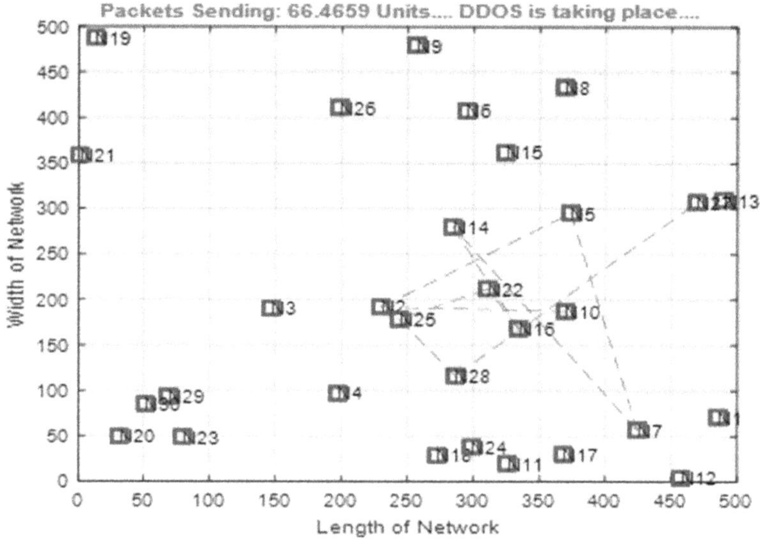

Figure 7.1 Network creation. (Sachdeva, 2018.)

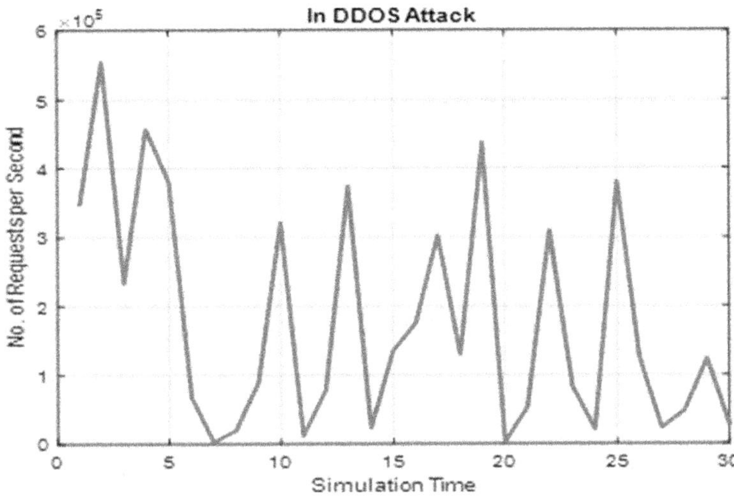

Figure 7.2 Number of requests per second. (Sachdeva, 2018.)

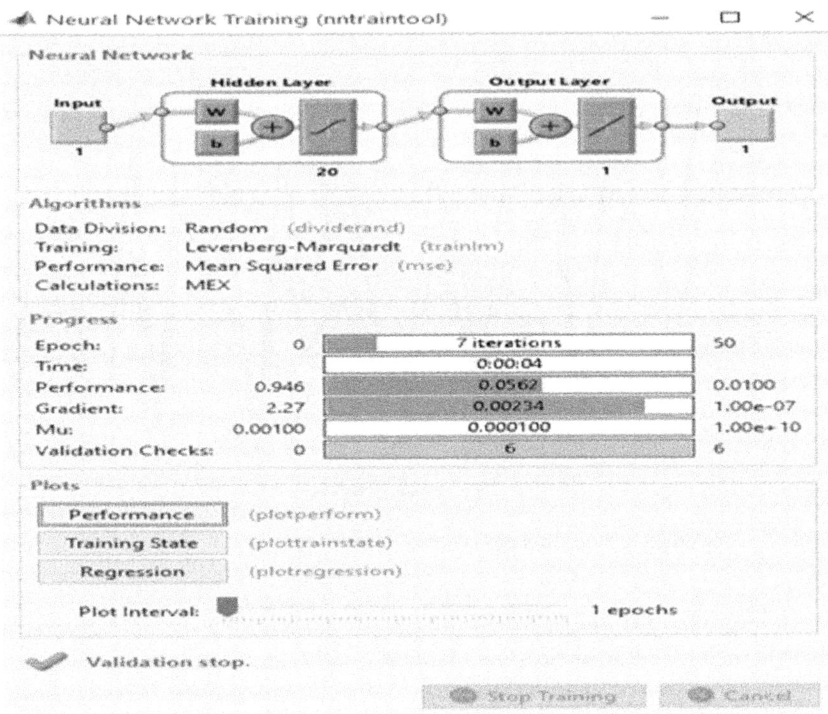

Figure 7.3 Network training. (Chuang, Liu, and Tsai, 2022.)

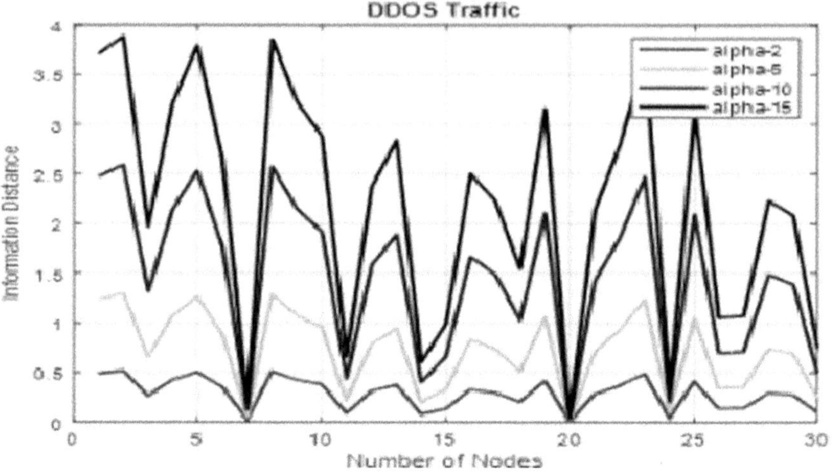

Figure 7.4 DDoS traffic classifications. (Sachdeva, 2018.)

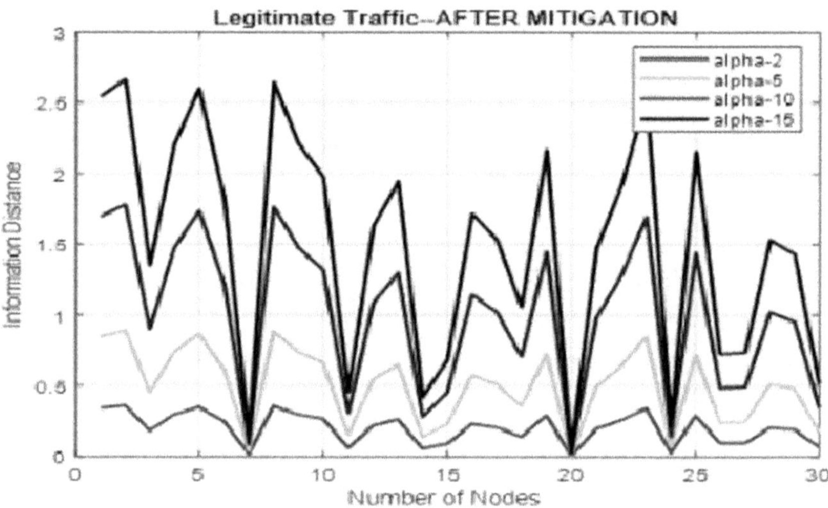

Figure 7.5 Legitimate traffic. (Sachdeva, 2018.)

traffic must be distinguished for the proper functioning of the network so that the network lifetime can be increased without any failures.

Figure 7.6 shows the overhead consumption which must be reduced for the efficient network lifetime. The overhead increases the load on the network nodes.

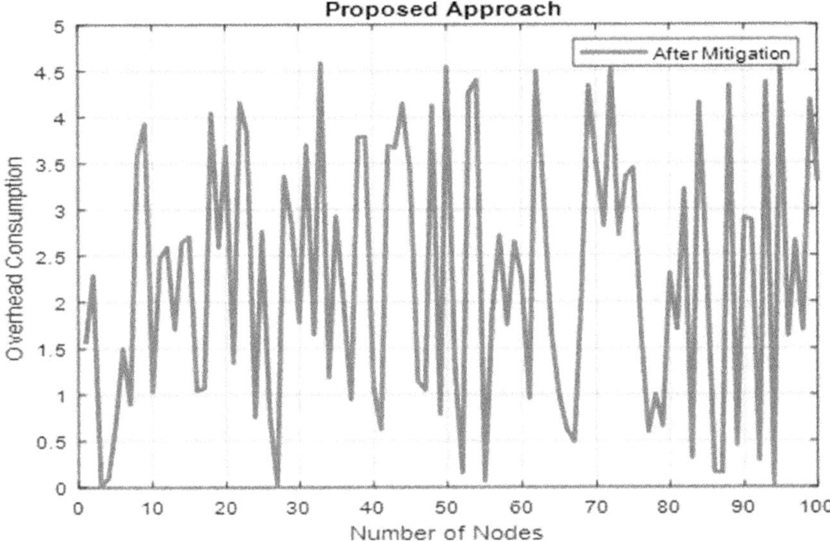

Figure 7.6 Overhead consumption. (Sachdeva, 2018.)

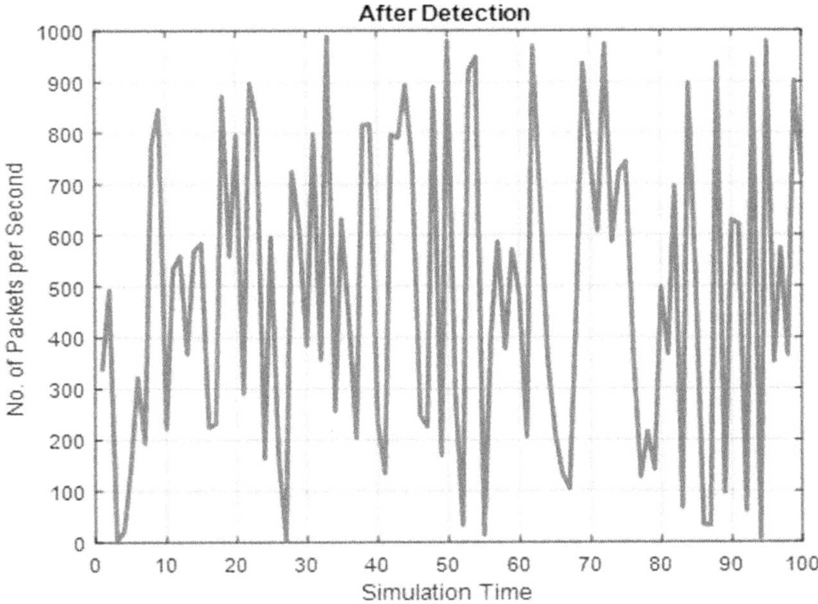

Figure 7.7 Number of packets per second. (Sachdeva, 2018.)

Figure 7.7 shows the number of packets among the network per second, which shows the high efficiency of the network in receiving the packets. This shows that the proposed approach can achieve high performance in the mitigation of the attack in the network, which will further reduce the overhead consumptions. The previous work uses a machine learning approach to differentiate legitimate traffic and DDoS traffic. The proposed work advances by effectively detecting both low-intensity and high-intensity DDoS attacks, mitigating these attacks, and significantly extending the network's lifespan.

7.7 CONCLUSION AND FUTURE SCOPE

In the proposed approach work is done to optimize the network by using a machine learning back propagation neural network, which hybridizes the optimization to achieve the performance evaluations in terms of mitigation effect. Due to the inherent constraints imposed by the node's finite resources, it becomes imperative for these nodes to engage in collaborative efforts. Multiple nodes can be assigned the responsibility of identifying a particular event. These nodes can work together in a network, with one node being designated to consolidate the sensor data from all other nodes in the network. This approach aims to minimize losses in the system and address uncertainties such SAS energy failures and network attacks. By doing so, the system can handle increased network loads, resulting in higher throughput and improved packet delivery rates with reduced errors. The suggested technique ultimately achieves a mitigation scenario for the DDoS assault, resulting in enhanced network performance. Future work will be to optimize the hybrid approach of the other optimization algorithms to reduce the uncertainties of achieving a lower error rate probability.

REFERENCES

Bawany, N.Z., Shamsi, J.A., and Salah, K. (2017). DDoS attack detection and mitigation using SDN: methods, practices, and solutions. *Arabian Journal for Science and Engineering*, 42, 425–441.

Behal, S., Kumar, K., and Sachdeva, M. (2018). Behal, S., et al. D-FAC: A novel /-Divergence based distributed DDoS defense system. *Journal of King Saud University – Computer and Information Sciences*. https://doi.org/10.1016/j.jks uci.2018.03.005

Chuang, H.M., Liu, F., and Tsai, C.H. (2022). Early detection of abnormal attacks in software-defined networking using machine learning approaches. *Symmetry*, 14(6), p. 1178.

Dhingra, A., and Sachdeva, M. (2021). Detection of denial of service using a cascaded multi-classifier. *International Journal of Computational Science and Engineering*, 24(4), 405–416.

Harithaa, R.B., and Vijayalakshmi, M. (2023, April). DDoS Attack Using Machine Learning: A Brief Survey. In *International Conference on Soft Computing for Security Applications* (pp. 829–840). Singapore: Springer Nature Singapore.

Korir, F., and Cheruiyot, W. (2022). A survey on security challenges in the current MANET routing protocols. *Global Journal of Engineering and Technology Advances*, 12(01), 078–091.

Liu, C., Gu, Z., and Wang, J. (2021). A hybrid intrusion detection system based on scalable K-means+ random forest and deep learning. *IEEE Access*, 9, 75729–75740.

Rasool, R.U., Ashraf, U., Ahmed, K. Wang, H., Rafique, W., and Anwar, Z. (2019). Cyberpulse: A machine learning based link flooding attack mitigation system for software defined networks. *IEEE Access*, 7, 34885–34899.

Reddy, K.G., and Thilagam, P.S. (2020). Naïve Bayes classifier to mitigate the DDoS attacks severity in ad-hoc networks. *International Journal of Communication Networks and Information Security*, 12(2), 221–226.

Sidhu, N., and Sachdeva, M. (2020). A comprehensive study of routing layer intrusions in zigbee based wireless sensor networks. *International Journal of Advanced Science and Technology*, 29(3), 514–524.

Zeng, F., Cheng, J., Cao, Z., Yang, Y., and Sheng, V.S. (2023, July). AcLGB: A Lightweight DDoS Attack Detection Method. In *International Conference on Information Science, Communication and Computing* (pp. 200–212). Singapore: Springer Nature Singapore.

Chapter 8

Role of artificial intelligence in healthcare

Neha Kaushal and Bhawna Kaushik

8.1 INTRODUCTION

The role of artificial intelligence in healthcare has been growing significantly. AI methods have shown to be quite successful in the medical field. The question of "Could artificial intelligence eventually take over the role of doctors in the future?" is another topic of intense debate. But it doesn't seem likely anytime soon. In certain areas, it can aid in making better healthcare decisions. Appropriate AI applications in the medical field are still being developed, helped along by the increasing accessibility of healthcare data and the quick development of big data analysis tools. When driven by relevant clinical questions, effective AI algorithms can potentially reveal valuable insights from large data sets, aiding in clinical decision-making. Healthcare professionals and organizations encounter various challenges such as shifting demographics, logistical needs, staffing shortages, and increasing rates of illness, alongside ongoing advancements in data technology and demand.

Artificial intelligence is increasingly being explored for various applications in clinical research and healthcare [1]. This research highlights the potential and benefits of AI-driven health solutions. Governments and innovation centers are collaborating to harness AI for medical advancements [2]. "The US Food and Drug Administration plans to increase the accessibility of clinical devices that utilize artificial intelligence." AI is expected to influence several key areas in healthcare delivery: patient follow-up, clinical decision support, healthcare organization, and medical interventions.

"The incorporation of cutting-edge technologies like cloud computing, the Internet of Things (IoT), and artificial intelligence" (AI) is transforming healthcare into a more efficient, effective, and personalized system. This approach allows individuals to manage their health more proactively through ongoing monitoring via mobile apps or wearable devices. Coupled with AI, this patient data can be transmitted to healthcare providers for

DOI: 10.1201/9781003518075-8

further analysis, facilitating early disease detection, ensuring treatment plans, and enhancing wellness screening.

8.2 LITERATURE REVIEW

"The benefits of artificial intelligence in healthcare have been widely explored in medical research." AI can utilize sophisticated algorithms to analyze large volumes of patient data, which can then enhance medical care. It has the potential to improve accuracy through learning and self-correction based on new data. AI systems that provide comprehensive clinical information from sources such as journals, textbooks, and medical procedures can assist healthcare providers in offering excellent patient care [3]. While diagnostic and therapeutic errors are an inherent part of human healthcare, AI systems can help mitigate these errors. Additionally, AI tools can analyze data from large patient populations to generate health risk alerts and predictions. The core of AI in healthcare involves data derived from medical activities such as screening, diagnosis, and treatment. This information encompasses demographics, medical histories, digital data from medical devices, clinical assessments, and laboratory tests and imaging. AI tools are generally categorized into two types: machine learning (ML) algorithms, processes that handle structured data, such as imaging and genomics [4], are complemented by natural language processing (NLP) techniques, which extract valuable information from unstructured data sources like clinical notes and medical literature. This integration helps to enhance and enrich structured medical data.

1. **Data Types in AI Research**

   AI research in medicine is expanding, but much of the focus remains on three primary disease categories: cardiovascular conditions, neurological disorders, and cancer [5]. This focus is expected given the high prevalence and significant mortality associated with these diseases. Early diagnosis of these conditions is crucial to prevent further health deterioration. AI systems are advancing techniques in imaging, genomics, electrophysiology (EP), and electronic medical records (EMR), which can enhance early detection and diagnosis of these critical diseases. Figure 8.1 shows different AI applications in healthcare.

2. The most common diseases are reviewed in the context of artificial intelligence (AI) research.

   The latest AI literature highlights the top ten types of diseases. Historically, AI advancements relied heavily on the expertise of medical specialists, but the field is now expanding rapidly. Recent AI

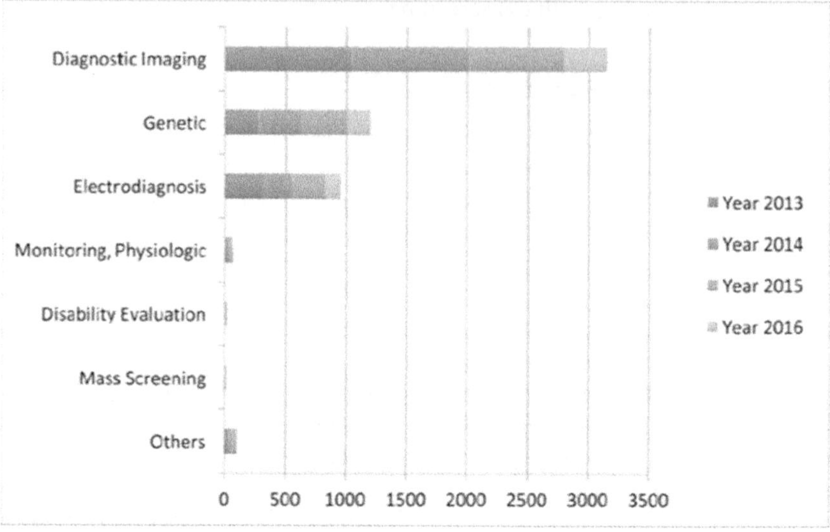

Figure 8.1 AI applications in healthcare.

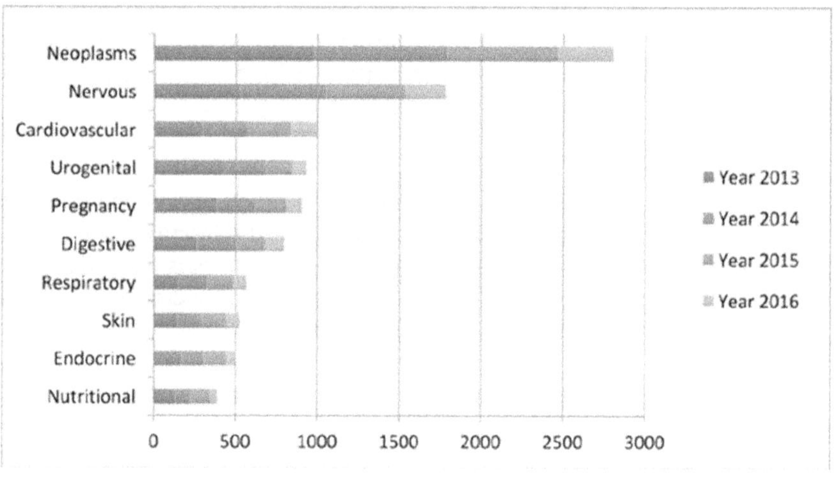

Figure 8.2 This image illustrates how artificial intelligence is applied in research of various kinds of diseases.

research has increasingly utilized machine learning techniques to uncover patterns in data, helping to elucidate complex relationships [6]. Figure 8.2 shows the major areas where researchers are applying AI for the early diagnosis and cure of several diseases. These AI

Table 8.1 How basic biomedical research supports the decisions taken by clinical experts

Basic biomedical research	Translational research	Clinical practice
Automated experiments	Biomarker discovery	Disease diagnosis
Automated data collection	Drug-target prioritization	Interpretation of patient genomes
Gene function annotation	Drug discovery	Treatment selection
Prediction of transcription factor binding sites	Drug repurposing	Automated surgery
Simulation of molecular dynamics	Prediction of chemical toxicity	Patient monitoring
Literature mining	Genetic variant annotation	Patient risk stratification for primary prevention

applications in healthcare are aiding clinical researchers in gaining a deeper understanding of patient conditions.

3. AI in medicine.

This provides a summary of existing and upcoming AI applications in the field of medicine. In assisted living, advanced robotics combined with AI technology improve the quality of life for seniors and individuals with disabilities. Human-machine interfaces (HMIs) enable people with disabilities to control wheelchairs and robotic devices without relying on conventional controllers or physical sensors, promoting increased independence. AI also enables visually impaired individuals to integrate into various fields, such as informatics and technology, using systems like RUDO, an "ambient intelligent system." Additionally, fall-detection systems help seniors avoid accidents, and biomedical researchers can utilize computational modelling assistants (CMAs) to transform relevant models into functional simulation tools. Here is a partial overview of current and anticipated AI applications in medicine (Table 8.1).

AI is revolutionizing the healthcare sector by assisting with data management, drug development, and various manual tasks. While AI brings numerous benefits, it also has its challenges. Its capacity to analyze data and enhance diagnostics supports routine administrative tasks, patient monitoring, and virtual consultations [2].

Since data is increasing at an exponential rate, training algorithms can become challenging quickly. Accessing some of the necessary data for model predictions can be challenging due to privacy issues. In the digital age, transitioning to artificial intelligence can be problematic, especially when patient safety is at stake. As the strategy demonstrates, we will first need evidence that AI will be successful.

Furthermore, given that investors and the healthcare sector are investing a sizable sum on this, will it be cost-effective?

8.3 OBSTACLES IN AI ADVANCEMENT

Artificial intelligence in healthcare faces several challenges, including the requirement for extensive data to effectively train neural networks and machine learning algorithms [7].

Nevertheless, it is rare that we obtain clear-cut or objective data. Information derived from disparate healthcare settings may be tainted by prejudice, noise, unbalanced medical data, missing details, etc. There's a chance the model developed using data from one institution won't translate to another. Consequently, scientists need to make sure that the information they gather accurately reflects the target patient population. One of the main challenges is that, while data is increasing rapidly, ensuring its accuracy at the decision-making stage remains crucial. Additionally, the responsibility of the AI system is a major concern, as incorrect information could potentially jeopardize a patient's life.

Trust is fundamental to the doctor-patient relationship. For effective treatment, patients need to have confidence in their doctor and believe in the efficacy of their care. Building this trust can be challenging when patients are unfamiliar with AI technologies. Trust is particularly important as AI contributes to patient care. Machine learning algorithms are created to examine data and generate insights. These systems use patient data and, in some cases, relevant medical outcomes to make predictions. Machine learning algorithms are typically divided into supervised and unsupervised learning categories. Supervised learning is commonly used for predictive modelling, while unsupervised learning is often applied for feature extraction. Figure 8.3 shows some of the major obstacles in the advancement of AI in healthcare.

4. Machine learning algorithm used in healthcare

In healthcare, machine learning algorithms are commonly utilized for a range of applications because they can process large volumes of data and uncover meaningful insights. Here are some prominent machine learning algorithms used in healthcare like Supervised Learning Algorithms:

- Support Vector Machines (SVM): SVMs are used for classification tasks such as disease prediction and diagnosis based on labelled data.
- Logistic Regression: Often used for predicting the likelihood of a particular outcome, such as patient mortality or readmission.
- Random Forests: Used for both classification and regression tasks, known for handling large datasets with many variables.

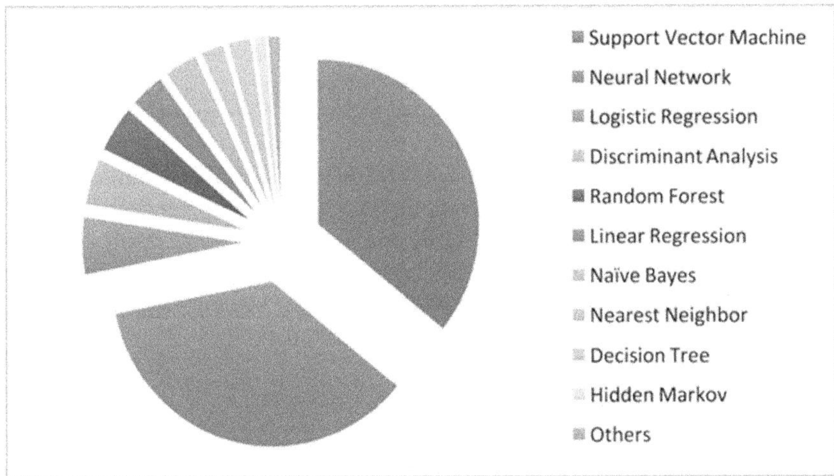

Figure 8.3 Obstacles in AI advancement.

2. Unsupervised Learning Algorithms:
   - Clustering Algorithms (e.g., K-means): Used to group patients or medical data into clusters based on similarities, aiding in patient segmentation or anomaly detection.
   - Principal Component Analysis (PCA): Reduces the dimensionality of large datasets, making it easier to analyze and interpret complex data.
3. Deep Learning Algorithms:
   - Convolutional Neural Networks (CNNs): Primarily used for image analysis tasks such as medical imaging (e.g., detecting tumors in CT scans) [8].
   - Recurrent Neural Networks (RNNs): Useful for analyzing sequential data, such as patient records over time, to predict outcomes or detect anomalies.
4. Natural Language Processing (NLP):
   - Algorithms such as Word Embeddings (e.g., Word2Vec) and Transformer Models (e.g., BERT): Used for processing and understanding textual data from medical records, clinical notes, and research literature.
5. Reinforcement Learning:
   - Emerging in healthcare for optimizing treatment plans and resource allocation based on patient outcomes and real-time data feedback.
   - Neural networks.

Artificial Neural Networks (ANNs) are the foundation of Artificial Intelligence. ANNs are able to find solutions to issues that are beyond the scope of human or mathematical comprehension. Figure 8.4 shows different algorithms used in various aspects of healthcare.

ANNs simulate human brain activity, including data processing and analysis. An ANN will learn on its own in the absence of a clear curriculum. An artificial neural network is made up of three types of layers: input, hidden, and output. Data is stored in the input layer neurons of the first layer and is moved to the second layer for additional processing. The result is output by the active neurons using the activation feature after they have passed through the hidden layer of the second layer [7]. The concealed layer could have many layers if the issue is more complicated.

6. The architecture of Artificial Neural Network

Deep learning refers to a more complex form of neural networks, characterized by its multi-layered architecture as shown in Figure 8.5. Deep learning techniques will analyze data in greater detail to uncover more complex non-linear patterns. Deep learning was used by the imaging researcher to emphasize how varied and expansive images are in general [8].

7. To gather information, a search was performed on PubMed to explore deep learning applications in healthcare and various disease categories a search was conducted on PubMed for deep learning applications in healthcare and disease categories.
8. The four most commonly utilized deep learning algorithms and their frequency of use.

Natural language interpretation textual forms of clinical data, including physical examination reports, clinical laboratory findings, and operation papers, are unstructured and unintelligible to computer programmers [9]. This involves discharge summaries where natural language processing (NLP) aims to extract relevant information from written texts to aid in treatment decisions. An NLP pipeline typically consists of text processing and categorization. The primary objective of this pipeline is to assist clinicians in monitoring side effects and making therapeutic decisions.

8.3.1 Artificial intelligence applications in stroke

Over the world, millions of individuals suffer from stroke. It ranks sixth in North America but is the leading cause of mortality in China. Therefore, research on stroke therapy and prevention is crucial [10].

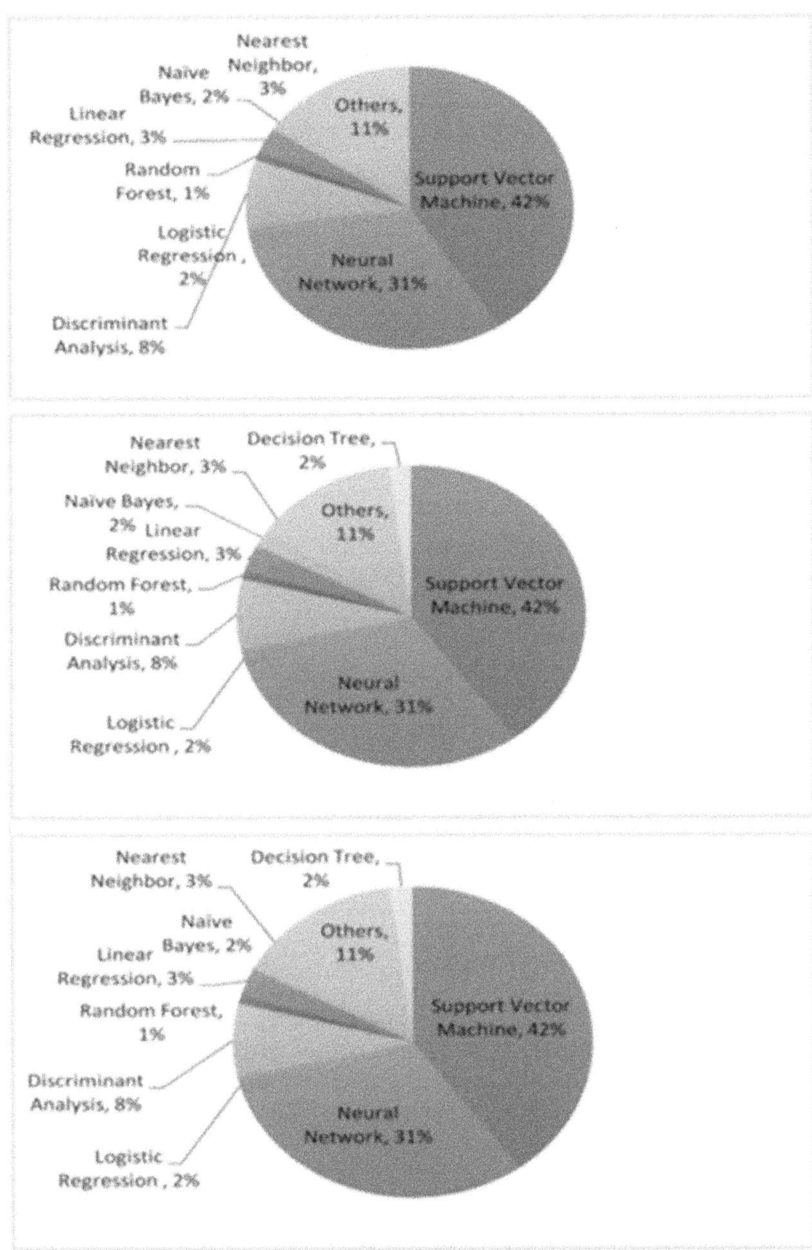

Figure 8.4 Human brain activity.

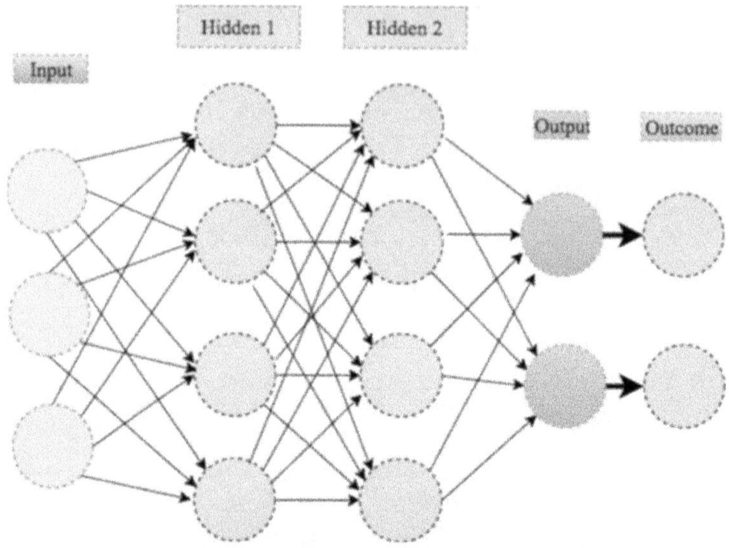

Figure 8.5 Architecture of Artificial Neural Network.

8.3.2 Early diagnosis and identification

The failure to identify early stroke symptoms meant that only a small number of patients could receive timely care. The detection procedure included stages for identifying human activity and detecting the onset of a stroke. A stroke warning is activated when a patient's movement significantly deviates from their typical pattern, and the patient is evaluated for care as quickly as feasible [11, 12].

8.3.3 Prognostic analysis and outcome prediction

Clinical mortality and stroke diagnosis are influenced by multiple factors. Machine learning approaches are superior to traditional methods when it comes to improving prediction accuracy [13]. To evaluate the data and enhance prediction accuracy, the authors used SVM and ANN [14]. Asadi et al. studied 107 individuals who underwent intra-arterial therapy for severe anterior or posterior circulation stroke [15]. Applying an enhanced algorithm outperformed previous techniques for predicting the 30-day death rate

8.4 CONCLUSION

We explored the reasons for implementing AI in healthcare, the various kinds of medical data analyzed by AI, and the prevalent disease categories where AI has been employed. Both machine learning and natural language processing (NLP), the two primary types of AI technologies, were thoroughly examined. In addition to traditional methods like SVM and neural networks, we explored a novel deep learning approach. Successful AI systems often include NLP for analyzing unstructured text, along with components for handling structured data like images, electrophysiological data, and genetic information.

In this context, the IBM Watson system stands out as a leader. This platform, which integrates both NLP and machine learning components, has demonstrated promising results in oncology. AI is anticipated to address increasingly complex and relevant clinical issues by utilizing extensive data and knowledge, thereby improving decision-making for stroke treatment. To ensure AI systems function effectively, they must continuously receive clinical trial data. Maintaining a steady data source is crucial for the ongoing advancement and refinement of an AI system that has been trained on historical information.

REFERENCES

[1] Jiang F, Jiang F, Hui Zhi, et al. Artificial intelligence in Healthcare: Past, present, and future. *Stroke and Vascular Neurology*, 2017; 2(2): 93–100. doi:10.1136/svn-2017-000101

[2] Patel VL, Shortliffe EH, Stefanelli M, et al. The coming age of artificial intelligence in medicine. *Artificial Intelligence in Medicine*, 2009; 46(1):5–17.

[3] Neill DB. Using artificial intelligence to improve hospital inpatient care. *IEEE Intelligent Systems*, 2013; 28:92–95.

[4] Gillies RJ, Kinahan PE, Hricak H. Radiomics: images are more than pictures, they are data. *Radiology*, 2016; 278(2):563–577.

[5] Esteva A, Kuprel B, Novoa RA, et al. Dermatologist-level classification of skin cancer with a deep neural network. *Nature*, 2017; 542:115–8.

[6] Bishop CM. *Pattern recognition and machine learning*, (Vol. 4, No. 4, p. 738), 2007. New York: Springer.

[7] Mirtskhulava L, Wong J, Al-Majeed S, et al. Artificial neural network model in stroke diagnosis, modelling and simulation. *2015 17th UKSim-AMSS International Conference on Modelling and Simulation (UKSim).* IEEE., 2015: 50–53.

[8] Ravi D, Wong C. Deep learning with health informatics. *IEEE Journal of Biomedical and Health Informatics*, 2017; 21(1): 4–21.

[9] Saenger AK, Christenson RH. Stroke biomarkers: progress and challenge for diagnosis, prognosis, differentiation, and treatment. *Clinical Chemistry*, 2010; 56:21–33

[10] Villar JR, Gonzalez S, Sendano J, et al. Improving human activity recognition and its application in early stroke diagnosis. *International Journal of Neural Systems*, 2015; 25:1450036.

[11] Bently P, Ganesalingam J, Jones AL, et al. Prediction of stroke thrombolysis outcome using CT brain machine learning. *Clinical*, 2014; 4:635–40.

[12] Lee D , Yoon, SN. Application of artificial intelligence-based technologies in the healthcare industry: Opportunities and challenges. *International Journal of Environmental Research and Public Health*, 1 January 2021; 18(1):271.

[13] Yu KH, Beam AL, Kohane IS, Artificial intelligence in healthcare. *Nature Biomedical Engineering*, 2018; 2:719–731.

[14] Rong G, Mendez A, Assic EB, Zhao B, Sawan M, Artificial intelligence in healthcare: Review and prediction case studies. *Engineering*, March 2020; 6(3):291–301. doi:10.1016/j.eng.2020.01.019

[15] Alemseged, F. (2021). Treatment and prognosis in posterior circulation ischaemic stroke (Doctoral dissertation, University of Melbourne).

Chapter 9

Intentions in the digital age

Paving the path to sustainable online insurance

Rekha Handa and Randeep Kaur

9.1 INTRODUCTION

ICT plays an important role in establishing a lasting equilibrium among individual progress as well as the environment as a whole, which is required for enduring economic growth (Souter et al., 2010). In numerous industries, technology for communication and information is transforming products, processes, organizations, and even business models. The digital transformation in numerous sectors has dramatically transformed the landscape of old processes, ushering in an exciting new age of efficiency, precision, and creativity. This trend is especially noticeable in the healthcare industry, where technology has transformed patient care, diagnosis, and treatment methods. Even technology has disrupted the insurance industry. Digital technologies are transforming the insurance business and encapsulating the insurance supply chain, increasing the industry's efficiency and defining insurance products (Stanković & Tomić, 2020). Insurance is a risk protection tool that helps in protection from uncertainties. The insurance industry helps in generating employment opportunities, reducing poverty, and thus helping in achieving various economic goals of the country. The insurance business plays a significant role in fostering sustainable financial and societal growth. The advancement in technology in the insurance industry is helping in achieving sustainable development goals, directly or indirectly. Insurance organizations may gradually switch to the insurance 4.0 model in order to improve resource conservation and promote sustainable economic endeavors (Nicoletti, 2021). Digital technology has the potential to improve the insurance industry's ability to offer solutions to a safe, secure, resilient, and sustainable society (Stankovic et al., 2020). Internet insurance services offer the ability to promote financial inclusion and minimize risks on an international scale. Customers' behavior, including both private policyholders and business customers, is critical to the longevity as well as the sustainability of internet-based insurance services. Further, artificial intelligence (AI) is establishing itself as a disruptive force in a variety of sectors, propelling tremendous improvements and altering established processes. AI's impact on healthcare has risen tremendously, altering several facets of the medical industry. AI systems can swiftly and correctly analyze large volumes of data, detecting behaviors and patterns that human physicians may miss. This skill is especially useful in diagnostics, whereby AI may help diagnose illnesses at an early stage, allowing for more prompt and effective treatments. Additionally, AI-powered prediction models can foresee patient outcomes, allowing healthcare professionals to make more educated treatment decisions. AI integration has also transformed multiple facets of the insurance sector, including underwriting and claims processing, as well as service to clients and identification of fraud. The imperative demand for accuracy and efficiency in insurance operations is being met by this technological advancement, which guarantees quick policy issuance, timely claim processing, and early fraud detection. Additionally, AI's capacity to evaluate big datasets and provide customized insurance solutions raises client happiness and loyalty. These developments lower operating costs, enhance risk management, and promote a more robust and customer-focused business model, all of which support the insurance industry's sustainability. Insurance companies can adjust to shifting market conditions and regulatory frameworks by utilizing AI, which will help them maintain long-term development and sustainability in the cutthroat digital era. Numerous studies have been conducted on the insurance industry's role in economic development and customer behavior towards insurance. Indian life insurance industry is the ninth largest life insurance industry in India (www.icicilombard.com). Insurance penetration and density are two indicators, among others, that are frequently used for assessing a country's insurance sector's level of development. Insurance penetration is defined as the proportion of insurance premium to GDP, whereas insurance density is determined as the premium to population ratio (per capita premium).

Insurance penetration in India in 2021-22 was 4.2%, the same as in 2020-21. Insurance penetration increased from 2.71% in 2001-02 to 5.2% in 2009-10 during the first ten years of insurance industry liberalization. Since then, the level of insurance penetration has dropped up until 2014-15, owing to a decline in life insurance penetration. However, insurance penetration began to increase again in 2015-16, reaching 4.20% in 2021-22. While life insurance penetration increased from 2.15% in 2001-02 to 3.2% in 2021-22, non-life insurance penetration increased from 0.56% to 1.0% during the same time period. Further life insurance companies have partnered with various web aggregators such as Easy Policy, Policy Bazaar etc. to increase insurance penetration and density of insurance services in India. Also, big insurance companies such as LIC, New India Assurance etc. have also introduced chatbots such as LIC Mitra, NYRA to improve the customer experience.

Quite a few research studies focus on the digital evolution of the insurance industry and the factors that contribute to the transition from traditional to online modes. This research investigates the drives that impact consumers' behavior and intentions towards using online insurance. The rationale behind this study is to know what factors drive the transition from traditional paperwork mode to online mode and how this transition affects the long-term health of the insurance industry to achieve the sustainability development goals (SDGs) in the economy.

9.2 LITERATURE REVIEW

The study has used a UTAUT2 model from social psychological theories as its theoretical base. The study has used the main four factors of the UTAUT2 model, which were integrated with two external variables, i.e., government support and perceived credibility, to predict the adoption of the information system for insurance services. Fig. 9.1 explains the structural relationships between the constructs.

A construct-based review of the literature has been done, which is as follows:

Performance Expectancy: The term "performance expectancy" refers to "the extent to which the person feels the usage of the technology would help him with task functioning" (Venkatesh et al., 2003). Performance expectancy has a significant relationship with behavior intention. This relationship has been supported by Tarhini et al. (2016) in the online banking context in Lebanon, Balakrishnan et al. (2022) in the chatbot-based services context, and Gu et al. (2021) in the e-health context in Pakistan. The proposition intended for this relationship is as follows:

H1: Performance expectancy has a favorable influence on behavioral intent to use online insurance services.

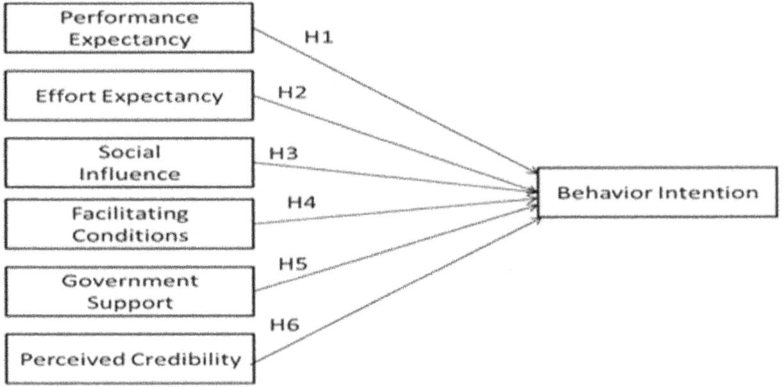

Figure 9.1 Theoretical Framework.

Effort Expectancy: "The extent of convenience attributed to the utilization of the system" (Venkatesh et al., 2003) is described as effort expectancy. Effort expectancy has a significant relationship with behavior intention, which has been supported by Bhatiasevi and Yoopetch (2015) and Merhi et al. (2019) in the mobile banking adoption context in Thailand and Britain, respectively. The hypothesis is as follows:

> *H2: Effort expectancy has a favorable association with the intention to use online insurance services.*

Social Influence: "The degree to which one believes how important others believe they ought to adopt the technology" (Venkatesh et al., 2003). The association of social influence with behavior intention is important. Yu et al. (2021) performed their research in the light of mobile-based health website use and supported this relationship through empirical testing. Chiu et al. (2012) supported this through their study on online sports lottery adoption in Taiwan. The proposition for this relationship is as follows:

> *H3: Social influence exhibits a significant association with behaviour and intention to utilize online insurance services.*

Facilitating Conditions: Facilitating conditions are defined as "the extent to which a person believes both a business and technological framework are present to facilitate system utilization" (Venkatesh et al., 2003). Facilitating conditions exhibit a significant relationship with behavior and intention. Chawla and Joshi (2019) conducted their study on mobile wallet adoption, and Zuiderwijk et al. (2015) conducted their study on acceptance of open data technologies. These studies support the relationship between facilitating conditions and behavior intention. The proposition for this relationship is as follows:

> *H4: Facilitating conditions exhibit a significant association with behaviour intent to use online insurance services.*

Government Support: "Government efforts to provide infrastructure and the regulatory environment for encouraging internet usage" (Tan & Teo, 2000). Government support has a significant relationship with behavior intention (Chi et al., 2015; Chong et al., 2010). The proposition for this relationship is as follows:

> *H5: Government support exhibits a significant association with the intention to use online insurance services.*

Perceived Credibility: It is referred to as an individual's personal trust in the system's ability to carry out a transaction safely while maintaining the confidentiality of their personal data (Mansour et al., 2016). Giao et al. (2020) and Jalal et al. (2011) both support the association in the context of internet banking and online banking, respectively. Perceived credibility has a significant relationship with behavior and intention. The hypothesis for this relationship is as follows:

> *H6: Perceived credibility exhibits a significant association with the intention to use online insurance.*

9.3 RESEARCH METHODOLOGY

A cross-sectional design was used in the current study. Data was collected using a survey instrument to assist in the attainment of the current study's aims. There are two components to the survey: the initial part includes Likert scale measurement items, and the second contains demographic information. The survey instrument involves 36 items on the scale. Measurement Scale items used for performance expectancy, social influence, effort expectancy, and facilitating conditions have been acquired from Venkatesh et al. (2003), and for government support, Nasri and Charfeddine (2012) and Chong et al. (2010) scales were used. The perceived credibility scale was adopted from Nasri and Charfeddine (2012). The questionnaire was first administered to five field experts to ensure the reliability of the scale and examine inefficiencies, and then a pilot survey with 100 respondents was conducted. After the pilot study, the questionnaire was improved according to the suggestions received from the experts and respondents. The five-point scale was employed, extending from "strong agree(1) to "strongly disagree" (5). The population of the study comprises those individuals who have either a "life or health insurance policy" and who have used any online service during the last year. Judgment sampling has been used to draw the sample. The sample size consists of 441 respondents from three districts of Punjab, namely "Amritsar, Jalandhar, and Ludhiana," representing Majha, Doaba, and the Malwa region, respectively. The data was collected in offline mode. Around 60.3% of total respondents were male, and 39.7% of respondents were female. The collected data was analyzed through structural equation modeling (SEM) in IBM AMOS. Structural equation modeling is a two-step process involving regression and factor analysis. Structural equation modeling is now a day's more preferred, specifically in studies like the adoption of IS/IT theories.

9.4 RESULTS AND DISCUSSION

The data was evaluated using Structured Equation Modeling (SEM). The fit indices of the measurement model are examined in the first stage. Further discriminant validity, reliability through average variance extraction, and composite reliability were also analyzed. Table 9.1 shows model fit index

Table 9.1 Model Fit Indices

Model fit indices	Measurement Model	Structural Model
Chi-square	689.111	712.066
Df	539	1.321
TLI	.983	.980
AGFI	.906	.905
CFI	.985	.982
NFI	.933	.931
RMSR	.028	.026
RMSEA	.025	.027

Notes: TLI- Tucker Lewis Indices, AGFI- Adjusted Goodness of Fit Indices, CFI- Comparative Fit Indices, NFI-Normed Fit Indices, RMSR- Root Mean Square Residual, RMSEA- Root Mean Square Error of Approximization and Computed using IBM AMOS.

Table 9.2 Composite Reliability, Average Variance Extracted, Discriminant Validity

	C.R.	A.V.E.	P.E.	E.E.	S.I.	P.C.	G.S.	B.I.	F.C.
P.E.	0.910	0.912	**0.818**						
E.E.	0.846	0.853	0.368***	**0.761**					
S.I.	0.909	0.910	0.400***	0.431***	**0.816**				
P.C.	0.916	0.918	0.368***	0.464***	0.492***	**0.803**			
G.S.	0.888	0.890	0.357***	0.428***	0.465***	0.524***	**0.754**		
B.I.	0.925	0.927	0.443***	0.331***	0.544***	0.587***	0.529***	**0.844**	
F.C.	0.874	0.878	0.331***	0.340***	0.391***	0.380***	0.294***	0.442***	**0.797**

Notes: PE: Performance Expectancy, EE: Effort Expectancy, SE: Social Influence, FC: facilitating Conditions, GS: Government Support, PC: Perceived Credibility, BI: Behavior Intention, Computed using IBM AMOS.

values for the measurement model (CFA). The finding indicates that each of the fit indices is within the acceptable range (Schermelleh-Engel et al., 2003). Further convergent validity was exhibited through two different measures, i.e., composite reliability and average variance extracted. Average variance extracted and composite reliability are more than 0.5 and 0.6, respectively shown in Table 9.2, and thus are within the acceptable range (Fornell et al., 1988). Discriminant validity shows that constructs are unique on their own, and Table 9.2 shows that there is no validity concern.

In the second stage, model fit indices are again examined in the structural model and presented in Table 9.1, which shows that each goodness of fit indices is according to threshold value. The structural relationships between the constructs were examined through beta coefficients and the p value. Table 9.3 shows that the results of the hypothesized paths between the latent variables were significant. Hypothesis 1 (β =.122, P<0.05) shows that performance expectation (PE) has a substantial effect on behavior intent

Table 9.3 Structural Relationships

Hypothesis	Path	Beta coefficient	P value	Result
H1	Performance Expectancy→ Behavior Intention	.122	***	Significant
H2	Effort Expectancy→ Behavior Intention	.145	.003	Significant
H3	Social Influence→ Behavior Intention	.156	***	Significant
H4	Facilitating Conditions→ Behavior Intention	.120	.005	Significant
H5	Government Support→ Behavior Intention	.186	***	Significant
H6	Perceived Credibility→ Behavior Intention	.320	***	Significant

towards using online insurance services. H2 (β =.145, P<0.05) indicates that effort expectancy (EE) influences behavioral intent to utilize online insurance services. H3 (β=.156, P<0.05) says that social influence has a noteworthy impact on behavior intending to utilize online insurance services.

H4 (β=.120, P<0.05) says that facilitating conditions have a significant positive influence on behavioral intent to utilize web insurance products. H5 (β=.186, P<0.05), government support has a significant positive impact on behavior intent to make use of online insurance services. H6 (β=.320, P<0.05), perceived credibility has a substantial influence on users' intent to utilize internet insurance services. As per the current study, all of the factors have a substantial impact on behavioral intent to utilize online insurance services.

Performance expectancy has been shown to have a noteworthy influence on behavior intended to utilize web insurance services. The finding reveals that system usefulness, in terms of saving time, efforts, and useful features, positively influences individuals' intention to switch from paper-based services to online mode. The result is in corroboration with various research studies (Balakrishnan et al., 2022; Galhena & Gunawardena, 2022; Gu et al., 2021; Tarhini et al., 2016). Further effort expectancy significantly impacts consumers' behavioral intention to use online insurance services. The findings indicate that website features such as ease of navigation and ease of use positively impact users' intent to use online services. The result is in congruence with previous research studies (Alduais & Al-Smadi, 2022; Bhatiasevi, 2016; Merhi et al., 2019). The intention to utilize internet insurance services is greatly influenced by social influence. Individuals believe that their choices for using online platforms, websites, and apps are influenced by their peers, family, and friends. The findings are supported by prior research studies (Chiu et al., 2012; Johar & Suhartanto, 2019). Users prefer using information technology over traditional paper-based services because facilities such as chat bot interactions and helpdesk facilities with less hassle are easily available on online platforms (Chawla & Joshi, 2019; Yu et al.,

2021; Zuiderwijk et al., 2015). Furthermore, government support turned out to have a strong favorable influence on behaviors and desires to use web insurance services. The findings show that initiatives by the government to achieve sustainable growth in the economy, such as digital drives and internet infrastructure, help form a positive intent to use online services. The results are in congruence with prior literature (Chi et al., 2015; Chong et al., 2010). Finally, perceived credibility was shown to have a strong favorable influence on behavior intending to utilize online insurance solutions. Robust security and privacy are the necessary features for online platforms. The present study shows that users believe that perceived credibility impacts their intent to use online insurance services. The findings are in corroboration with previous literature (Giao et al., 2020; Jalal et al., 2011; Tarhini et al., 2016). A study by NASSCOM on online insurance adoption shows that 88% of 2000+respondents prefer using digital and hybrid models for insurance services.

9.5 IMPLICATIONS

The present study has practical implications for the insurance industry. The findings show performance expectancy as a considerable construct of behavior intention, and users give significant attention to the usefulness of the online platforms. Thus, insurance companies can use this finding and must focus on building useful features for the various online platforms, such as websites, apps, etc. Additionally, findings indicate that effort expectancy turned out to be significant in influencing users' intent to use information systems for insurance services. Thus, the findings give useful insights to insurance companies, and companies can work on improving the complexities of using computer technology. Moreover, findings revealed that individuals are easily influenced by the people around them. The insurance companies can use these findings and ask social media influencers to market their products to enhance their customer base. Thus, the objectives of sustainability can also be achieved. The findings of the present study are helpful for insurance providers as they can provide better security features, such as encryption and demo options, on the website, thus resulting in greater customer satisfaction. Switching from a paper-based traditional mode to an online mode for using insurance services can help achieve sustainability development goals. This can be done with government support by educating individuals and creating awareness among them regarding sustainable insurance options.

9.6 LIMITATION AND FUTURE SCOPE

The present study only focused on the Punjab region; thus, the results of the study may not be globally applicable. The research focused on a quantitative approach; a qualitative approach could have a better result. The present study has used UTAUT2 as a conceptual framework only; it can be integrated with other technology adoption models to predict the adoption of information systems. Further variables like trust and risk can be used in combination with a theoretical model from the social-psychological domain.

9.7 CONCLUSION

Technology has immense influence on users' behavior towards insurance services. Users these days prefer easy and sustainable solutions for their needs. Artificial intelligence such as chatbots in the front end helps the users have a pleasurable experience, while the use of artificial intelligence for claim processing in the back end also proves beneficial for insurance companies to satisfy their customers. Even the artificial intelligence in the medical field proves useful in detecting fraud, making the right diagnosis as physicians, and handling large amounts of patient data. Privacy and security are key concerns that motivate or discourage users' use of technology for insurance services. Thus the advent of artificial intelligence as a part of digital transformation is useful and necessary in healthcare and insurance.

REFERENCES

Alduais, F., & Al-Smadi, M. O. (2022). Intention to use E-Payments from the perspective of the Unified Theory of Acceptance and Use of Technology (UTAUT): Evidence from Yemen. *Economies, 10*(10), 259. https://doi.org/10.3390/economies10100259

Balakrishnan, J., Abed, S. S., & Jones, P. (2022). Technological Forecasting & Social Change The role of meta-UTAUT factors, perceived anthropomorphism, perceived intelligence, and social self-efficacy in chatbot-based services? *Technological Forecasting & Social Change, 180*(December 2021), 121692. https://doi.org/10.1016/j.techfore.2022.121692

Bhatiasevi, V. (2016). An extended UTAUT model to explain the adoption of mobile banking. *Information Development, 32*(4), 799–814. https://doi.org/10.1177/0266666915570764

Bhatiasevi, V. and Yoopetch, C. (2015). The determinants of intention to use electronic booking among young users in Thailand. *Journal of Hospitality and Tourism Management, 23*, 1–11.

Chawla, D., & Joshi, H. (2019). Consumer attitude and intention to adopt mobile wallet in India – An empirical study. *International Journal of Bank Marketing, 37*(7), 1590–618. https://doi.org/10.1108/IJBM-09-2018-0256

Chi, L., Kazmi, A., Hasnain, S., Hai, L. C., Hasnain, S., & Kazmi, A. (2015). Munich Personal RePEc Archive Dynamic Support of Government in Online Shopping. 66027. https://doi.org/10.5539/ass.v11n22p1

Chiu, Y. T. H., Lee, W. I., Liu, C. C., & Liu, L. Y. (2012). Internet Lottery Commerce: An Integrated View of Online Sport Lottery Adoption. *Journal of Internet Commerce, 11*(1), 68–80. https://doi.org/10.1080/15332861.2012.650990

Chong, A. Y. L., Ooi, K. B., Lin, B., & Tan, B. I. (2010). Online banking adoption: An empirical analysis. *International Journal of Bank Marketing*, 28(4), 267–287. https://doi.org/10.1108/02652321011054963

Fornell, C., Larcker, D., Perreault, W., & Anderson, C. (1988). Structural Equation Modeling in Practice: A Review and Recommended Two-Step Approach. *Psychological Bulletin*, 103(3), 411–423.

Galhena, B. L., & Gunawardena, K. A. T. P. P. (2022). Drivers of Intention to Use Internet Banking: Unified Theory of Acceptance and Use of Technology Perspective. *Wayamba Journal of Management*, 13(1), 181. https://doi.org/10.4038/wjm.v13i1.7558

Giao, H. N. K., Vuong, B. N., Tung, D. D., & Quan, T. N. (2020). A Model of Factors Influencing Behavioral Intention to Use Internet Banking and the Moderating Role of Anxiety: Evidence from Vietnam. *WSEAS Transactions on Business and Economics*, 18, 10–20. https://doi.org/10.37394/23207.2021.18.2

Gu, D., Khan, S., Khan, I. U., Khan, S. U., Xie, Y., Li, X., & Zhang, G. (2021). Assessing the Adoption of e-Health Technology in a Developing Country: An Extension of the UTAUT Model. *SAGE Open*, 11(3), 21582440211027565. https://doi.org/10.1177/21582440211027565

Jalal, A., Marzooq, J., & Nabi, H. A. (2011). Evaluating the Impacts of Online Banking Factors on Motivating the Process of E-banking. *Journal of Management and Sustainability*, 1(1), 32–42. https://doi.org/10.5539/jms.v1n1p32

Johar, R. S., & Suhartanto, D. (2019). The Adoption of Online Internet Banking in Islamic Banking Industry. *IOP Conference Series: Materials Science and Engineering*, 662(3). https://doi.org/10.1088/1757-899X/662/3/032032

Mansour, I. H. F., Eljelly, A. M. A., & Abdullah, A. M. A. (2016). Consumers' attitude towards e-banking services in Islamic banks: the case of Sudan. *Review of International Business and Strategy*, 26(2), 244–260. https://doi.org/10.1108/RIBS-02-2014-0024

Merhi, M., Hone, K., & Tarhini, A. (2019). Technology in Society A cross-cultural study of the intention to use mobile banking between Lebanese and British consumers: Extending UTAUT2 with security, privacy and trust. *Technology in Society*, 59(June), 101151. https://doi.org/10.1016/j.techsoc.2019.101151

Nasri, W., & Charfeddine, L. (2012). Factors affecting the adoption of Internet banking in Tunisia: An integration theory of acceptance model and theory of planned behavior. *Journal of High Technology Management Research*, 23(1), 1–14. https://doi.org/10.1016/j.hitech.2012.03.001

Nicoletti, B. (2021). Benefits and challenges of digital transformation. *Insurance 4.0: Benefits and Challenges of Digital Transformation*, 361–387.

Schermelleh-Engel, K., Moosbrugger, H., & Müller, H. (2003). Evaluating the fit of structural equation models: Tests of significance and descriptive goodness-of-fit measures. *MPR-Online*, 8(May), 23–74.

Souter, D., MacLean, D., Akoh, B. and Creech, H. (2010). ICTs, the Internet and Sustainable Development: Towards a new paradigm. IISD. Canada. Retrieved from https://coilink.org/20.500.12592/c2hbr7 on 01 Dec 2024. COI: 20.500.12592/c2hbr7

Stanković, J. Z., & Tomić, J. (2020). Digitalization and Sustainability-Opportunities and Challenges for Insurance Industry. *Economic Archive*, 2, 43–57.

Tan, M. and Teo, T. S. (2000). Factors influencing the adoption of Internet banking. *Journal of the Association for Information Systems*, 1(1), 5.

Tarhini, A., El-Masri, M., Ali, M., & Serrano, A. (2016). Extending the utaut model to understand the customers' acceptance and use of internet banking in Lebanon a structural equation modeling approach. *Information Technology and People*, 29(4), 830–849. https://doi.org/10.1108/ITP-02-2014-0034

Venkatesh, V., Morris, M. G., & Davis, G. B. (2003). User acceptance of information technology: towards a unified view. *MIS Quarterly*, 27(3), 425–478. https://doi.org/10.1016/j.inoche.2016.03.015

Yu, C. W., Chao, C. M., Chang, C. F., Chen, R. J., Chen, P. C., & Liu, Y. X. (2021). Exploring Behavioral Intention to Use a Mobile Health Education Website: An Extension of the UTAUT 2 Model. *SAGE Open*, 11(4), 21582440211055721. https://doi.org/10.1177/21582440211055721

Zuiderwijk, A., Janssen, M., & Dwivedi, Y. K. (2015). Acceptance and use predictors of open data technologies: Drawing upon the unified theory of acceptance and use of technology. *Government Information Quarterly*, 32(4), 429–440. https://doi.org/10.1016/j.giq.2015.09.005

Chapter 10

Enhancing anatomical education through artificial intelligence

Integrating security and ethical dimensions – a comprehensive review

Sonal Talreja

10.1 INTRODUCTION: BACKGROUND AND DRIVING FORCES

The foundation of medical professionals' education is clinical anatomy, which provides the fundamental information needed for clinical practice. There is an increasing interest in using artificial intelligence (AI) to anatomical education in order to improve and transform learning experiences in this age of rapid technology innovation. In the context of contemporary literature, artificial intelligence (AI) is defined as computer systems that perform tasks that conventionally require human intelligence, make predictions and decisions based on data analysis, and identify meaningful patterns—all without explicit guidance beyond basic programming [1, 2].

Clinical settings have long been using AI for a variety of purposes, including detection and diagnostic tools, patient triage decision-support systems, patient anomaly identification, intraoperative feedback, and clinical note and text summarization [3]. There is growing interest every year in the use of AI systems and algorithms in clinical education [4–10]. Figure 10.1 illustrates the increasing quantity of papers from PubMed published in the field of "Artificial intelligence + Clinical education" since 2004. It is worth noting that the majority of the papers indexed (about 80%) were published between 2020 and 2024. As the field of education develops, academics are attempting to use cutting-edge AI methods—such as data mining and deep learning—to address challenging problems and personalize instruction for each student.

This chapter explores the state of AI applications today, with a focus on anatomy teaching. It looks at cutting-edge technology like 3D anatomical modeling, adaptive learning platforms, AI-driven evaluation tools, and virtual anatomy dissection software. It also discusses the difficulties and moral issues surrounding the incorporation of AI into educational systems and offers suggestions for their successful application.

This chapter seeks to shed light on the revolutionary potential of artificial intelligence (AI) in anatomy education by combining a wide range of

   DOI: 10.1201/9781003518075-10

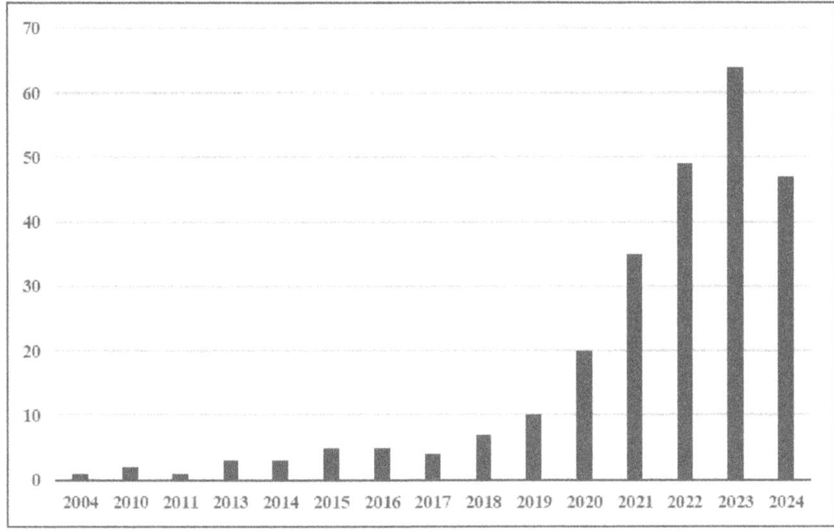

Figure 10.1 Number of Papers with the keywords "AI" + "Clinical Education" in the last twenty years. (PubMed.)

previously published works and practical examples. It emphasizes the significant influence AI can have on how anatomical knowledge is taught and learned, and it promotes continued study and innovation in this area. In the end, this investigation highlights the need for the medical education community to adopt AI-driven innovations in order to promote better learning outcomes and better equip upcoming medical professionals for the intricacies of clinical practice. Figure 10.2 shows possible applications of AI in the field of Anatomical Education.

10.2 AI APPLICATIONS IN ANATOMICAL EDUCATION

10.2.1 Virtual Anatomy Dissection Software

Artificial Intelligence-driven Virtual Anatomy Dissection Software presents a strong substitute for conventional cadaveric dissection. These digital platforms generate highly realistic, interactive, and configurable virtual anatomical models with the use of AI algorithms. Students can dissect tissues, examine anatomical structures in three dimensions, and see intricate linkages with never-before-seen clarity. For instance, learners can interactively study anatomical structures and functions with the help of the Visible Body's Human Anatomy Atlas [11], which uses AI algorithms to create realistic 3D models of the human body. It is a subscription-based

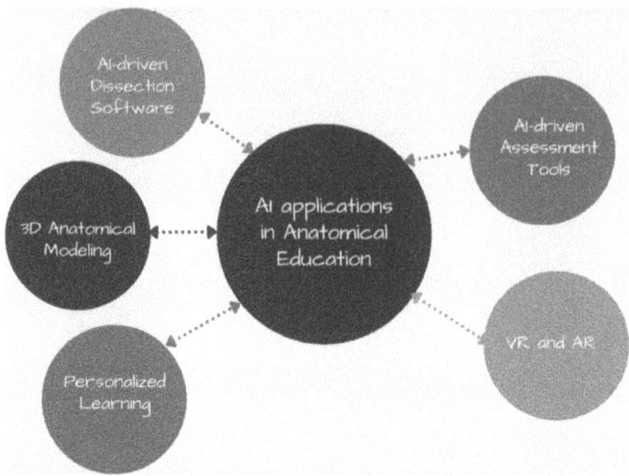

Figure 10.2 Applications of AI in Anatomical Education.

educational resource that helps physicians and health science students expand and improve their understanding of human anatomy. This software includes quizzes, patient education films, cadaver lab simulations, comparisons to diagnostic imaging, and thousands of 3D models of gross anatomy and microanatomy [12].

Anatomy Studio performs 3D reconstruction of anatomic structures by contour drawing on 2D images of actual cross-sections (cryosections), combining tablet sketching with MR-based viewing [13]. The interactive tablet surface facilitates natural drawing, but compared to typical desktop methods, the 3D representation delivers a better sense of the reconstructed information. Moreover, Anatomy Studio can be interacted with by allowing users to navigate around the slices in the MR display with mid-air motions. We can leverage the benefits of both interaction paradigms when we combine mid-air input with interactive surfaces. This is because multi-modal interface research has shown that the synergistic combination of both modality and interactive surface should likely surpass the drawbacks of each one separately. Anatomy Studio also allows multiple experts to work together, facilitating communication and displaying in real-time the changes each expert has made to the shapes [13].

10.2.2 3D Anatomical Modeling

The development of complex three-dimensional anatomical models based on data from medical imaging tests like computed tomography (CT) and magnetic resonance imaging (MRI) has advanced dramatically with the application of AI algorithms in medical education. With the unmatched ability to manipulate in real time, these AI-powered models let medical professionals and students explore anatomical variances, practice complex surgical techniques, and understand spatial relationships in a dynamic way. For example, the Stanford 3DQ Lab uses AI to create 3D anatomical models that are patient-specific and intended for both teaching and surgical planning. This method enhances learning by enabling a deeper comprehension of intricate anatomical structures and diseases [14].

Furthermore, a variety of platforms, including PCs, mobile apps, and standalone interactive workstations like Anatomage and Touch of Life [15], provide access to digital 3D models of anatomical systems. The use of these digital tools at study workstations and in gross anatomy laboratories greatly lessens the need for tangible anatomical models or printed atlases. Through instantaneous and interactive access to comprehensive anatomical information, this digital transformation improves the educational process by bringing anatomical material right to the dissecting table. The capacity of digital 3D models to be temporally altered is a noteworthy benefit that enables instructors and students to exhibit and investigate variations in anatomical structures over time. These can include changes brought on by aging, the effects of illnesses or accidents, and differences in functional mechanics. Students obtain a thorough grasp of the dynamic nature of human anatomy by viewing these temporal changes [16].

10.2.3 Personalized learning

Personalized learning experiences are provided by AI-powered adaptive learning platforms, which take into account the unique traits, interests, and abilities of each student. By analyzing student data and identifying areas of strength and weakness, these systems use machine learning algorithms to customize instructional content. To maximize learning results, adaptive learning platforms can provide scaffolded learning experiences, targeted remediation, and real-time feedback. One illustration is the adaptive learning platform from McGraw-Hill called SmartBook. This platform uses artificial intelligence (AI) algorithms to dynamically modify the level of content according to the success of each learner, giving each student a tailored learning route.

A dynamic approach to learning is provided by adaptive artificial intelligence, which is especially helpful in complicated domains like human anatomy. There are many benefits to teaching anatomy with adaptive learning modules. The ability to learn at one's own pace is the primary benefit, as it is essential for comprehending the complexities of anatomical structures and functions. These platforms' adaptive features guarantee that education is tailored to each student's needs while highlighting their strengths. This individualized method greatly improves knowledge retention while also increasing student enthusiasm and engagement [17].

Moreover, adaptive learning platforms offer an environment for learning that is more dynamic and interesting. These platforms keep students actively involved in their education by continuously adapting to their demands, which improves the effectiveness and enjoyment of the learning process. This is especially crucial for topics like anatomy, where future clinical practice requires a profound and nuanced grasp.

All things considered, AI-driven adaptive learning systems mark a substantial breakthrough in educational technology. Through individualized, focused education and instantaneous feedback, these platforms facilitate students' acquisition of a more thorough and durable comprehension of intricate subjects. Technology is expected to be applied in anatomy education and other sectors more and more as it develops, providing even more advanced tools and techniques for improving learning results [17].

10.2.4 Virtual reality (VR) and augmented reality (AR)

By combining AI with these technologies, anatomy education has been transformed and is now possible thanks to immersive and dynamic learning environments. With the use of these state-of-the-art tools, students can practice procedural skills in a risk-free setting, participate in virtual dissections, and navigate through anatomical structures in simulated clinical scenarios. By enabling students to engage directly with anatomical models, VR and AR go beyond simple observation and promote experiential learning, leading to a greater comprehension of intricate structures and their roles.

The HoloAnatomy program at Case Western Reserve University [18], which uses Microsoft's HoloLens AR technology to produce holographic anatomical models, is one prominent example of this integration. With the help of these dynamic models, students may explore and manipulate anatomical components in real time, offering a hands-on learning opportunity that goes beyond conventional teaching techniques. Virtual reality (VR) and augmented reality (AR) technologies provide unmatched opportunities for simulation-based training, immersive learning, and group-based educational experiences by submerging students in a three-dimensional virtual environment.

The use of VR and AR in anatomy education signifies a paradigm change in the approaches used in instruction. By facilitating interactive investigation, these tools not only improve student engagement and retention but also encourage active learning. VR and AR help students better prepare for the challenges of real-world healthcare settings by closing the knowledge gap between theory and practice by replicating realistic clinical scenarios and offering opportunity for hands-on experience.

Furthermore, by enabling several users to engage with the same virtual models at once, VR and AR promote collaborative learning. This improves peer-to-peer learning, collaboration, and communication skills, which benefits everyone's educational experience. The incorporation of virtual reality (VR) and augmented reality (AR) into anatomy education holds great potential to transform the way students engage with and learn about anatomical concepts, thereby influencing the course of medical education and practice in the future [19].

10.2.5 AI-driven Assessment Tools

By using AI algorithms, assessment procedures in anatomy education can be significantly improved. Grading can be automated, real-time feedback can be given, and learner performance data can be analyzed. These evaluation instruments are able to assess student performance in a variety of areas, including procedural skills, clinical reasoning, and anatomical knowledge. This allows teachers to identify areas that need work and adjust their instructional strategies accordingly. For example, the Learning Catalytics platform [20] uses artificial intelligence (AI) to assess student replies to quiz questions in real-time, giving teachers important information on how engaged and knowledgeable their students are.

Additionally, AI-driven evaluation tools provide insightful information about student performance, allowing teachers to pinpoint areas in which pupils consistently fail. The basis for curriculum creation and instructional design is provided by this data, which guarantees that teaching tools and materials are carefully crafted to meet the individual needs of students. Additionally, by helping students become more self-aware of their learning progress and areas for growth, the platform's metacognitive assessment tools promote the development of lifelong learning abilities [17].

10.3 CHALLENGES AND CONSIDERATIONS

Although there are many advantages of integrating AI into anatomy teaching, there are also issues and concerns that need to be taken into account. In the field of biomedical imaging, there are possibilities and challenges. For anatomical imaging techniques, these include lower radiation doses and faster acquisition rates. The creation of algorithms should take into account variations in imaging parameters (such as slice thickness, in-plane resolution, etc.) as they may have a significant impact on image analysis and were not covered in the discussion. Furthermore, the massive volume of imaging data created necessitates a substantial demand for informatics in order to store, transmit, analyze, and interpret the data automatically. This is the foundation for the application of big data science to better utilization and diagnosis [21].

10.3.1 Technical Challenges

To guarantee the efficacy and dependability of AI-powered teaching resources, a number of technological issues pertaining to the integration of

AI into clinical anatomy education must be resolved. It takes a multidisciplinary team with knowledge of computer science, AI, and educational technology to develop these products. But it's possible that educators lack the knowledge and resources needed to properly develop, deploy, and manage AI-driven learning environments. This underscores the necessity of professional development initiatives and cooperative efforts among educators, technologists, and AI specialists to mitigate this disparity and guarantee the triumphant incorporation of AI in the teaching of clinical anatomy.

Furthermore, there are several technical obstacles to overcome in order to guarantee the precision, dependability, and scalability of AI algorithms in educational contexts. To properly assess and understand complex anatomical structures, AI algorithms need to be trained on vast quantities of anatomical data. Finding and selecting high-quality anatomical data, however, can be challenging; in order to obtain pertinent information, cooperation with medical institutes and organizations is necessary. Furthermore, constant research and development activities are required to update and improve AI algorithms in order to stay up with advances in medical knowledge and technology.

Concerns over the moral use of AI technology are also raised by the incorporation of AI into clinical anatomy instruction. Teachers need to make sure that AI-powered learning resources follow moral principles and protect patient confidentiality and privacy. This entails putting strong data security measures in place to safeguard private medical data and getting patients' and students' informed consent before allowing them to engage in AI-powered learning activities. Ensuring that AI technologies are utilized responsibly and ethically in clinical anatomy instruction demands close oversight and cooperation with regulatory organizations and ethics committees.

To summarize, a number of technological obstacles must be removed before AI-powered teaching resources may reach their full potential in clinical anatomy education. Through interdisciplinary collaboration, continuous research and development, and ethical oversight, educators can effectively utilize artificial intelligence (AI) to improve clinical anatomy education and better equip upcoming medical professionals for the intricacies of clinical practice [22, 23].

10.3.2 Ethical Considerations

In order to ensure the ethical and responsible use of these tools, educators must address the considerable ethical considerations raised by the incorporation of AI technology in clinical anatomy education. Data privacy, algorithmic bias, and equal access are the three main ethical issues.

Data privacy: Artificial intelligence (AI)-powered instructional systems frequently rely on enormous volumes of data, including private medical records. Teachers need to make sure that these resources respect learners' right to privacy and comply with stringent data privacy laws. To protect sensitive data, this calls for the use of strong data encryption, access controls, and anonymization methods. Before collecting and using students' data, educators must have their informed consent. They also need to be transparent about how students' data will be used and shared.

Algorithmic Bias: When AI algorithms are trained on data that contains prejudices, they may unintentionally reinforce these biases, producing unfair results and widening already existing gaps. Algorithmic bias in clinical anatomy education may lead to inaccurate or misleading anatomical models, diagnostic tools, or instructional materials. By routinely reviewing AI algorithms, diversifying training datasets, and putting fairness-aware machine learning approaches into practice, educators may be proactive in detecting and reducing algorithmic biases. Teachers should also assess AI-powered learning resources thoroughly to make sure they support inclusion, equity, and diversity in anatomy instruction.

Equitable Access: To guarantee that all students have the chance to profit from these technologies, access to educational resources driven by AI should be equal. On the other hand, differences in access to digital resources and technology could make already-existing educational inequities worse. By providing sufficient infrastructure and resources, providing training and support for students from underserved communities, and taking into account the accessibility needs of diverse students during the design and implementation process, educators can promote equitable access to AI-powered educational tools.

Apart from tackling these moral dilemmas, teachers are essential in encouraging students' digital literacy and ethical consciousness. Teachers should include ethical issues, algorithmic bias, and data privacy into their curricula so that students may employ AI technology in their professional activity and critically assess them. Educators may guarantee that AI-powered teaching tools improve learning outcomes while respecting ethical principles and advancing social justice in clinical anatomy education by cultivating a culture of ethical awareness and responsible usage of AI [24].

10.3.3 Integration into Curricula

To enable the successful deployment of AI in curriculum, educators and institutions need to solve a number of issues. Among these difficulties are:

Curriculum Redesign: Including AI into current curricula necessitates a thorough revision of the teaching resources, educational activities, and evaluation techniques. In order to integrate AI-driven educational tools into course content, this approach includes determining how AI can improve learning outcomes and changing learning objectives and course content. Redesigning a curriculum can take a lot of time and resources, therefore faculty members and curriculum architects must carefully plan and coordinate the process.

Faculty Development: Teachers might not have the information and abilities needed to successfully incorporate AI into their lesson plans. In order to give teachers the guidance and assistance they need to integrate AI-driven learning resources into their classes, promote interactive learning, and using AI technology to evaluate students' learning outcomes, faculty development programs are crucial. However, institutional support and specialized resources are needed to carry out faculty development projects.

Institutional Support: In order to successfully integrate AI into curricula, institutions must offer the infrastructure, resources, and support required. To enable AI-driven instructional tools, this entails making investments in hardware upgrades, software licenses, and technological infrastructure. Institutions must also set rules and regulations for the moral application of AI in teaching, as well as give staff members and instructors continuous technical support.

Ongoing Support and Training: To guarantee that teachers can successfully integrate AI-driven teaching resources into their lesson plans, ongoing support and training are crucial. For the purpose of exchanging ideas and sharing best practices, educators require access to cooperative communities of practice, technological support, and continual training opportunities. Ongoing training and assistance, however, necessitate consistent funding and dedication from institutions.

All things considered, incorporating AI into the curriculum presents serious obstacles that need to be overcome even if it also presents exciting chances to improve teaching and learning results. Through meticulous planning, faculty development, institutional support, and continuous

Table 10.1 Challenges faced due to integration of AI in anatomy teachings

Challenges	Issues Faced	Possible Resolution
Technical	Lack of knowledge or resources Precision, dependability, scalability of AI algorithms Finding and selecting high quality anatomical data Constant updation/improvement AI algorithms	Interdisciplinary collaboration, continuous research & development, ethical oversight
Ethical	Data privacy Algorithmic Bias Equitable Access	Cultivating culture of ethical awareness and responsible usage of AI
Integration into Curricula	Curriculum redesign Faculty development Institutional Support Ongoing support and training	Meticulous planning, faculty development, institutional support, continuous training and assistance

training and assistance, educators can effectively incorporate artificial intelligence (AI) into their curricula and equip students for the opportunities and difficulties presented by the digital era [25].

This can be well summarized as in Table 10.1.

10.4 FUTURE DIRECTIONS

10.4.1 Personalized Learning Pathways

The ability of AI algorithms to customize educational experiences to each learner's requirements, interests, and career goals in the context of personalized learning pathways signifies a significant change in the way that education is provided and experienced. Here's more information to clarify this:

Customized to Meet the Needs of Each Learner: Large volumes of learner data, such as performance metrics, learning preferences, and styles, can be analyzed by AI algorithms. AI can create individualized learning pathways that are tailored to the specific requirements of every student by using this data. With recommendations for particular topics or concepts depending on their competence levels, for instance, learners can concentrate their efforts on areas where they most need assistance.

Tailored Educational Materials: Personalized learning routes give students access to tailored educational materials that match their interests and learning objectives. With the use of artificial intelligence (AI), learning resources such as articles, videos, interactive simulations, and tests may be carefully selected based on the interests and professional goals of each learner. With this tailored approach, students are guaranteed to interact with knowledge that is pertinent, interesting, and significant to their educational path.

Real-time progress tracking tools and customized feedback are two features that AI-driven personalized learning platforms can offer to students. Students get quick feedback on their work, enabling them to pinpoint their areas of strength and growth. Furthermore, progress tracking tools let students keep tabs on their progress toward learning goals, celebrate their successes, and modify their approach to learning as needed.

Enhanced Motivation and Learner Engagement: By giving students the freedom to direct their own education, personalized learning pathways promote higher levels of motivation and learner engagement. Learners are more likely to feel motivated and committed in their academic endeavors when they have control over the speed, substance, and direction of their education. To increase student motivation and engagement, AI algorithms can also include gamification components like leaderboards, prizes, and badges.

Growth of Self-Directed Learning abilities: Self-directed learning abilities like goal planning, time management, and introspection are encouraged via personalized learning paths. AI-driven learning platforms promote independence and autonomy by letting students choose how to proceed through the course material. In order to establish the groundwork for both professional competence and lifelong learning, learners must be able to recognize their own learning requirements, set reasonable goals, and take proactive measures to attain them.

In conclusion, AI-powered personalized learning paths have the potential to completely transform education by offering customized learning experiences that are catered to the unique requirements and preferences of every student. Personalized learning pathways boost learner engagement, motivation, and self-directed learning skills by providing focused feedback, progress monitoring features, and customized instructional content. This eventually improves learning outcomes and professional competency.

10.4.2 Lifelong Learning Platforms

By providing chances for ongoing education that is customized to each learner's needs and career path, AI-powered lifelong learning platforms have the potential to completely transform the professional development of healthcare professionals. Here's more information on how these platforms can help with continuing professional development and skill enhancement:

Just-in-Time Educational Materials: AI algorithms are used by platforms for lifelong learning to provide healthcare workers with timely and relevant learning materials. These platforms offer real-time access to the most recent knowledge and best practices, enabling professionals to stay informed and up to date despite the rapid changes in the medical sector. These developments may include new treatment procedures, revised guidelines, or emerging research discoveries.

Peer Collaboration Facilitation: Online communities, discussion boards, and cooperative projects are some of the ways that lifelong learning platforms encourage communication and cooperation between medical professionals. AI algorithms can facilitate peer-to-peer learning and mentorship opportunities by bringing together experts with comparable hobbies, specializations, or learning objectives. This cooperative setting encourages the sharing of knowledge, insights, and experiences, which enhances education and develops a culture of ongoing development.

Possibilities for Continued Skills Development: Throughout the course of a medical profession, a variety of learning opportunities are provided by platforms for lifetime learning, which help with continued skill development. Through case-based learning modules, virtual reality experiences, interactive simulations, and virtual patient contacts, these platforms offer practitioners practical learning opportunities where they can hone their clinical abilities without taking any risks.

Healthcare professionals can use lifetime learning platforms to stay up to date with the latest developments, best practices, and emerging trends in their area. In order to fill in knowledge gaps or meet new demands, AI algorithms can evaluate learner data to pinpoint areas that require skill development and provide pertinent learning opportunities. Healthcare workers may guarantee superior patient care and adjust to changing demands in the delivery of healthcare by remaining knowledgeable and proactive in their learning process.

Assistance for Professional Development: The development of healthcare professionals' careers and their professional progress are greatly aided by platforms for lifelong learning. These platforms help professionals grow their skill sets, gain more knowledge, and progress in their jobs by providing possibilities for credentialing and certification, as well as individualized learning pathways and career development resources. In addition to helping professionals become better practitioners, ongoing investment in professional development also improves patient outcomes and organizational success.

In conclusion, AI-driven platforms for lifelong learning have the potential to enable healthcare workers to pursue lifelong learning, keep up with new developments, and further their careers. Through the provision of timely learning materials, peer cooperation, and opportunities for continuous skill enhancement, these platforms guarantee that medical professionals maintain their competence, self-assurance, and ability to provide patients with high-quality care throughout their career path.

10.4.3 Interdisciplinary Collaboration

The effective integration of AI into anatomy education depends on interdisciplinary collaboration since it brings together a variety of viewpoints and areas of knowledge to promote innovation and excellence in teaching and learning. Here's more information about how industrial partners, educators, developers, and healthcare professionals may work together to improve the way artificial intelligence is used in anatomy education:

Teachers: Teachers offer priceless insights into instructional design, curriculum development, and pedagogy. Their partnership with engineers and healthcare experts guarantees that AI-powered learning resources meet learning goals, accommodate a range of learning preferences, and encourage learners to take an active role in their education. Teachers are also essential in assessing how well AI technologies improve learning outcomes and offer feedback for continuous improvement.

Technologists: These professionals are skilled in software development, AI, and UX design. Their partnership with educators enables the creation of AI-powered learning resources that make use of state-of-the-art technology to produce engaging and dynamic learning environments. In order to create user-friendly interfaces, incorporate AI algorithms for individualized learning pathways, and guarantee smooth connection with current educational platforms and systems, technologists collaborate closely with educators.

Healthcare Workers: The clinical knowledge and practical understanding that healthcare workers provide to the field of anatomy education is invaluable. Their partnership with educators and tech experts guarantees that AI-powered learning resources take into account the intricacies of clinical practice, cover pertinent clinical scenarios, and provide content that is supported by research. Moreover, in order to guarantee that AI-generated anatomical models and simulations adhere to professional standards and best practices, healthcare practitioners must validate the clinical relevance and accuracy of these models.

Industry Partners: Industry partners facilitate the creation and application of AI-driven educational products by contributing resources, knowledge, and technical infrastructure. In order to enhance the area of anatomy education, educators and technologists can access cutting-edge technologies, data analytics skills, and research funding through collaborative research efforts with industry partners. Industry partners also provide information about user preferences, market trends, and industry standards that helps shape the creation of scalable and commercially successful artificial intelligence (AI) tools for anatomy teaching.

Research efforts: Innovation and knowledge exchange in anatomical education are fueled by collaborative research efforts including educators,

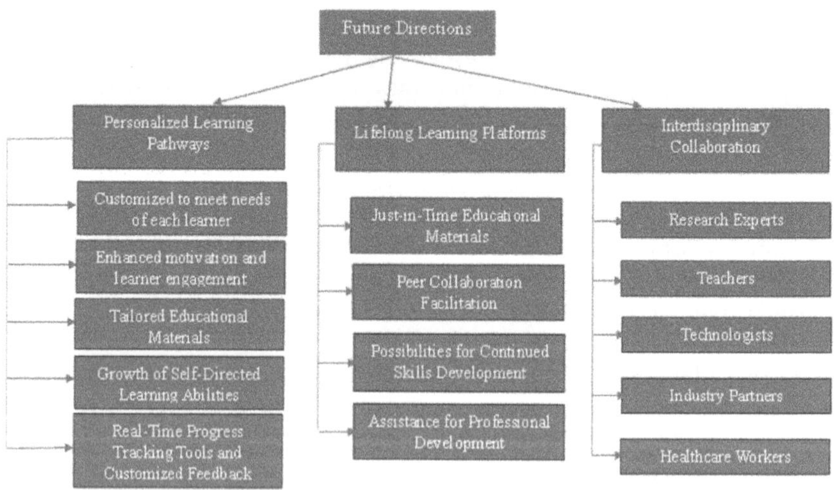

Figure 10.3 Possible Future Directions.

technologists, healthcare practitioners, and industry partners. These programs build a culture of ongoing learning and development, enable interdisciplinary cooperation, and add to the body of research demonstrating the efficacy of AI-powered teaching resources. The results of joint investigations can influence standards, guidelines, and best practices for integrating AI into anatomy education, so influencing the future course of the profession.

To sum up, progressing the integration of AI into anatomical education requires interdisciplinary collaboration between educators, technologists, healthcare practitioners, and industrial partners. Collaboration fosters innovation, excellence, and ultimately improves the teaching and learning process in anatomy education by utilizing group knowledge, resources, and ideas. Figure 10.3 shows the possible future directions in the field of anatomy education with the integration of AI.

10.5 CONCLUSION

The use of artificial intelligence (AI) into medical education is a revolutionary development in the field of anatomy, with the potential to improve patient care by raising the standard of teaching. Educators may create dynamic, tailored, and immersive learning experiences that not only engage learners but also foster clinical proficiency and deep comprehension by leveraging AI-powered technology. AI-driven platforms have the ability to completely transform the way anatomy is taught, learned, and used in clinical settings, which has enormous benefits.

An extensive review of artificial intelligence's (AI) current status and potential future applications in anatomy teaching is given in this book chapter. Through a thorough examination, it explains the various applications of AI, highlights the difficulties and factors to be taken into account when implementing it, and suggests methods for optimizing AI's usefulness in medical education. This chapter becomes an invaluable resource for academics, educators, and medical professionals interested in using artificial intelligence (AI) to improve anatomy training and develop medical knowledge because of its multidisciplinary approach and practical insights.

Most importantly, the chapter gives a road map for maximizing artificial intelligence in medical education. By outlining tactics for efficient application and optimization, it enables academics, researchers, and medical professionals to make use of AI's transformative potential. The chapter emphasizes the collaborative effort necessary to realize AI's promise in anatomy education by promoting cross-disciplinary collaboration and ongoing innovation.

In summary, this book chapter illuminates the way toward a future in which artificial intelligence (AI) drives significant breakthroughs in medical practice and anatomy teaching. It not only informs but also inspires action with its combination of multidisciplinary ideas and practical advice, calling on stakeholders to set out on a path of discovery, creativity, and change in the quest for excellence in medical education and healthcare delivery.

REFERENCES

[1]   N. Selwyn, and B. G. Cordoba, "Australian public understandings of artificial intelligence", *Ai & Society*, vol. 37, no. 4, pp. 1645–1662, 2022.

[2]   R. Tanwar, S. Bhatia, V. Sapra, and N. J. Ahuja, *Artificial Intelligence and Machine Learning: An Intelligent Perspective of Emerging Technologies.* CRC Press, 2023.

[3]   A. Banerjee, C. Chakraborty, A. Kumar, and D. Biswas, "Emerging trends in IoT and big data analytics for biomedical and health care technologies", in Valentina Emilia Balas, Vijender Kumar Solanki, Raghvendra Kumar and Manju Khari (eds.), *Handbook of data science approaches for biomedical engineering*, 2020, pp. 121–152. Elsevier.

[4]   G. B. Auffenberg, K. R. Ghani, S. Ramani, E. Usoro, B. Denton, C. Rogers, B. Stockton, D. C. Miller, and K. Singh, "askMUSIC: Leveraging a Clinical Registry to Develop a New Machine Learning Model to Inform Patients of Prostate Cancer Treatments Chosen by Similar Men", European Urology, vol. 75, no. 6, pp. 901–907, 2019.

[5]   A. Offiah, J. Hume, I. Bamsey, H. Jenkinson, and B. Lings, "ELECTRICA: ELEctronic knowledge base for Clinical care, Teaching and Research In Child Abuse", *Pediatric Radiology*, vol. 41, no. 11, pp. 1433–9, 2011.

[6]   A. Maier, M. Hartung, M. Abovsky, K. Adamowicz, G. D. Bader, S. Baier, D. B. Blumenthal, J. Chen, M. L. Elkjaer, C. Garcia-Hernandez, M. Helmy, M. Hoffmann, I. Jurisica, M. Kotlyar, O. Lazareva, H. Levi, M. List, S. Lobentanzer, J. Loscalzo, N. Malod-Dognin, Q. Manz, J. Matschinske, M. Mee, M. Oubounyt, C. Pastrello, A. R. Pico, R. T. Pillich, J. M. Poschenrieder, D. Pratt, N. Pržulj, S. Sadegh, J. Saez-Rodriguez, S. Sarkar, G. Shaked, R. Shamir, N. Trummer, U. Turhan, R. S. Wang, O. Zolotareva, and J. Baumbach, "Drugst.One – a plug-and-play solution for online systems medicine and network-based drug repurposing", *Nucleic Acids Research*, vol. 52, pp. W481–W488, 2024.

[7]   J. Stourac, S. Borko, R. T. Khan, P. Pokorna, A. Dobias, J. Planas-Iglesias, S. Mazurenko, G. Pinto, V. Szotkowska, J. Sterba, O. Slaby, J. Damborsky, and D. Bednar, "PredictONCO: A web tool supporting decision-making in precision oncology by extending the bioinformatics predictions with advanced computing and machine learning", *Briefings in Bioinformatics*, vol. 25, pp. bbad441, 2023.

[8]   F. Ranchon, S. Chanoine, S. Lambert-Lacroix, J. L. Bosson, A. Moreau-Gaudry, and P. Bedouch, "Development of artificial intelligence powered apps and tools for clinical pharmacy services: A systematic review", *International Journal of Medical Informatics*, vol. 172, pp. 104983, 2023.

[9]   Z. Q. P. Ng, L. Y. J. Ling, H. S. J. Chew, and Y. Lau, "The role of artificial intelligence in enhancing clinical nursing care: A scoping review", *Journal of Nursing Management*, vol. 30, no. 8, pp. 3654–3674, 2022.

[10] E. Morrow, T. Zidaru, F. Ross, C. Mason, K. D. Patel, M. Ream, and R. Stockley, "Artificial intelligence technologies and compassion in healthcare: A systematic scoping review", *Frontiers in Psychology*, vol. 13, pp. 971044, 2023.

[11] Visible Body Suite [Online], Available: www.visiblebody.com/anatomy-and-physiology-apps/vb-suite

[12] G. Schwartzman, and P. Ramamurti, "Visible body human anatomy atlas: Innovative anatomy learning", *Journal of Digital Imaging*, vol. 34, no. 5, pp. 1328–1330, 2021.

[13] E. R. Zorzal, M. Sousa, D. Mendes, R. K. dos Anjos, D. Medeiros, S. F. Paulo, P. Rodrigues, J. J. Mendes, V. Delmas, J. F. Uhl, J. Mogorrón, J. A. Jorge, and D. S. Lopes, "Anatomy studio: A tool for virtual dissection through augmented 3D reconstruction", *Computers & Graphics*, vol. 85, pp. 74–84, 2019.

[14] Y. AbouHashem, M. Dayal, S. Savanah, and G. Štrkalj, "The application of 3D printing in anatomy education", *Medical Education Online*, vol. 20, no. 1, pp. 29847, 2015.

[15] Anatomage Table – 3D Anatomy [Online], Available: https://anatomage.com/table/

[16] J. R. Fredieu, J. Kerbo, M. Herron, R. Klatte, and M. Cooke, "Anatomical models: A digital revolution", *Medical Science Educator*, vol. 25, pp. 183–194, 2015.

[17] M. Vertemati, G. V. Zuccotti, and M. Porrini, "Enhancing Anatomy Education Through Flipped Classroom and Adaptive Learning. A Pilot Project on Liver Anatomy", Preprints, 2024010218, 2024.

[18] Case Western Reserve University, HoloAnatomy® Software Suite [Online], Available: https://case.edu/holoanatomy/

[19] E. D. Fajrianti, S. Sukaridhoto, M. U. H. A. Rasyid, B. E. Suwito, R. P. N. Budiarti, I. A. A. Hafidz, N. A. Satrio, and A. L. Haz, "Application of augmented intelligence technology with human body tracking for human anatomy education", *IJIET: International Journal of Information and Education Technology*, vol. 12, no. 6, pp. 476–484, 2022.

[20] Pearson, Learning Catalytics [Online], Available: www.pearson.com/en-ca/higher-education/products-services/learning-catalytics.html

[21] A. S. Panayides, A. Amini, N. D. Filipovic, A. Sharma, S. A. Tsaftaris, A. Young, D. Foran, N. Do, S. Golemati, T. Kurc, K. Huang, K. S. Nikita, B. P. Veasey, M. Zervakis, J. H. Saltz, and C. S. Pattichis, "AI in medical imaging informatics: current challenges and future directions", *IEEE Journal of Biomedical and Health Informatics*, vol. 24, no. 7, pp. 1837–1857, 2022.

[22] M. D. Lazarus, M. Truong, P. Douglas, and N. Selwyn, "Artificial intelligence and clinical anatomical education: Promises and perils", *Anatomical Science Education*, vol. 17, pp. 249–262, 2022.

[23] M. P. Recht, M. Dewey, K. Dreyer, C. Langlotz, W. Niessen, B. Prainsack, and J. J. Smith, "Integrating artificial intelligence into the clinical practice of radiology: challenges and recommendations", *European Radiology*, vol. 30, pp. 3576–3584, 2020.

[24] M. Ienca, and K. Ignatiadis, "Artificial Intelligence in Clinical Neuroscience: Methodological and Ethical Challenges", *AJOB Neuroscience*, vol. 11, no. 2, pp. 77–87, 2020.

[25] B. Guimarães, L. Dourado, S. Tsisar, J. M. Diniz, M. D. Madeira, and M. A. Ferreira, "Rethinking Anatomy: How to Overcome Challenges of Medical Education's Evolution", *Acta Med Port*, vol. 30, pp. 134–140, 2017.

Chapter 11

A comprehensive exploration of sentiment analysis methods for social media data using Python

Jayadharshini Periasamy, Santhiya Saminathan, Abinaya Nagarajan, Abirami Thiyagarajan, Samyuktha Kathirvel, and Srimathi Elango

11.1 INTRODUCTION

In brand new interconnected international landscape, social media structures have come to be vibrant arenas in which people from numerous backgrounds converge to proportion their thoughts, reviews, and reviews on an array of topics. This consistent glide of person-generated content affords a goldmine of facts that gives priceless insights into public sentiment, purchaser conduct, and rising tendencies. On the center of harnessing this wealth of statistics lies sentiment evaluation, a powerful method that permits the extraction of significant insights from the sizable troves of textual content statistics located on social media systems. On this bankruptcy, we embark on a comprehensive exploration of sentiment evaluation strategies in particular those tailor-made for social media records, employing the versatile programming language Python. To lay a stable basis, we start by delving into the essential standards underpinning sentiment analysis. Knowing how the essence of sentiment analysis is critical as it forms the bedrock upon which greater advanced strategies are built. We elucidate the numerous procedures to sentiment evaluation, starting from rule-based totally methods to machine, getting to know algorithms, presenting readers with a nuanced information of the methodologies at their disposal.

Shifting ahead, we delve into the sensible components of records preparation, a crucial step inside the sentiment evaluation pipeline. This includes loading raw facts from social media platforms, preprocessing textual content to put off noise and inappropriate data, and extracting applicable capabilities using installed models, which include the Bag of phrases version. Sentiment analysis helps understand user-generated data on social media, which allows insight into public opinion and trends [1–3]. It is necessary for business firms to keep tabs on customer feedback, thereby enhance services and strategize in accordance with the sentiments of the people [4].

Through distinctive causes and hands-on examples, readers benefit from a skill ability in preparing social media information for sentiment evaluation

DOI: 10.1201/9781003518075-11

responsibilities. With the solid expertise of information education under our belt, we pivot inside the direction of superior techniques aimed in the direction of improving the accuracy and effectiveness of sentiment analysis on social media records. We explore the combination of phrase embeddings, sentiment lexicons, and complicated deep learning fashions together with recurrent neural networks (RNNs) and convolutional neural networks (CNNs). With the aid of leveraging these advanced methodologies, readers gain insights into the way to address the inherent worrying situations of sentiment assessment inside the dynamic and nuanced landscape of social media.

Moreover, the bankruptcy addresses the vital trouble of area version, presenting insights into strategies for customizing sentiment evaluation fashions to precise social media domain names. It emphasizes the importance of adapting fashions to various linguistic styles, terminologies, and cultural nuances established in precise social media systems. Throughout the chapter, readers are guided with code examples and implementation records, leveraging famous Python libraries including NLTK, scikit-observe, gensim, and TensorFlow. Those practical demonstrations facilitate the assimilation of sentiment evaluation techniques, enabling analysts and researchers to discover deeper insights into public opinion, sentiment trends, and rising subjects for the duration of severe social media structures.

Furthermore, we delve into strategies for domain adaptation, recognizing that sentiment evaluation models have to be adaptable to the specific characteristics and nuances of different social media domains. Via strategies such as transfer studying and domain-particular fine-tuning, readers discover ways to tailor sentiment evaluation fashions to fit the precise necessities of various social media platforms, ensuring strong performance throughout specific contexts. Armed with this understanding, analysts and researchers can gain unencumbered deeper insights into public opinion, sentiment developments, and emerging subjects, empowering them to make informed decisions in today's rapidly evolving digital panorama.

11.2 FEATURE ENGINEERING TECHNIQUES

In addition to elucidating the foundational Bag of Words model, the chapter delves into a spectrum of advanced feature engineering techniques tailored to enhance the accuracy and effectiveness of sentiment analysis on social media data. Advanced techniques such as TF-IDF and n-grams are widely used for enhancing sentiment analysis models [5], [7]. Word embeddings, which represent words as dense, low-dimensional vectors, have further improved the contextual understanding of sentiment [4], [8]. These methods have significantly contributed to capturing sentiment nuances in textual data.

11.2.1 TF-IDF (Term Frequency-Inverse Document Frequency)

TF-IDF is a widely-used method that is going past simple phrase counts by weighing the significance of phrases in files relative to their frequency throughout the whole corpus. This technique addresses the restrictions of Bag of phrases by way of assigning better weights to phrases which might be frequent in a file but rare throughout the whole corpus, hence highlighting terms which might be more discriminative and informative for sentiment evaluation. By means of incorporating TF-IDF capabilities, sentiment evaluation models can seize the essence of social media posts, discern sentiment nuances and identify key expressions that affect the overall sentiment.

11.2.2 N-grams

In addition to individual words, n-grams capture sequences of adjacent words within text data, ranging from bi-grams (sequences of two words) to higher-order n-grams. By considering sequences of words rather than just isolated terms, n-grams provide a means to preserve crucial contextual information, capturing nuances in language usage and syntactic structures present in social media discourse. For example, phrases like "not good" or "very happy" may convey sentiment meanings that are not apparent when analyzing individual words in isolation. By incorporating n-grams as features, sentiment analysis models can better grasp the subtleties of sentiment expression, leading to more accurate and nuanced sentiment predictions.

11.2.3 Word embeddings

Phrase embeddings represent words as dense, low-dimensional vectors in a continuous vector area, in which semantically comparable words are positioned toward each different word. Via encoding semantic relationships and contextual nuances, word embeddings provide a more nuanced representation of textual content compared to standard one-hot encoding or Bag of phrases. This technique permits sentiment evaluation models to seize semantic similarities and infer sentiment from contextual cues, thereby enhancing accuracy, mainly in situations where words with similar meanings but one-of-a-kind bureaucracy are used.

Through comprehensive examples and practical insights, readers are ready with the information and tools that are important to adeptly manipulate text facts, optimize feature representations, and refine sentiment evaluation models for heightened accuracy and overall performance inside the dynamic realm of social media analytics.

11.3 HANDLING IMBALANCED DATA

Dealing with imbalanced records is an important factor of sentiment evaluation, particularly inside the context of social media, in which sure sentiments may dominate the discourse while others are relatively rare. Important when dealing with imbalanced data sets is in sentiment analysis tasks since specific sentiments dominate the social media texts. Oversampling and class weighting are among the used strategies that have been widely deployed so far [5], [7]. Failure to cope with magnificence imbalance can result in biased models that perform poorly on minority instructions, undermining the overall accuracy and reliability of sentiment evaluation outcomes. In this section, we explore numerous strategies to mitigate the challenges posed via imbalanced statistics:

11.3.1 Resampling techniques

Over-sampling: This entails growing the variety of instances inside the minority class by way of replicating current samples or generating synthetic samples using techniques like SMOTE (artificial Minority Over-sampling method). Under-sampling: Conversely, underneath-sampling reduces the number of instances in the general public class by means of randomly getting rid of samples till a balanced distribution is done.

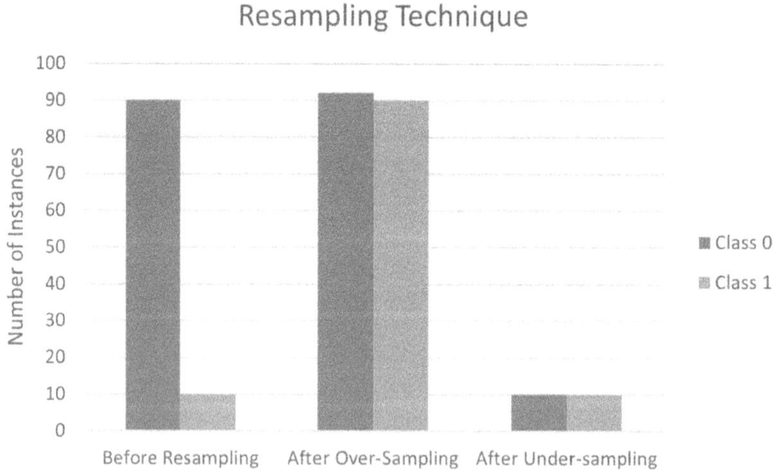

Figure 11.1 A chart comparing different resampling techniques (over-sampling, under-sampling) and their impact on class distribution in a dataset.

11.3.2 Class weighting

Assigning higher weights to minority class samples during model training can be an effective strategy to penalize misclassifications of these instances. Most machine learning libraries offer options for setting class weights, which can be adjusted inversely proportional to class frequencies.

11.3.3 Ensemble methods

Ensemble learning techniques such as Bagging and Boosting can be employed with base learners trained on balanced subsets of data or with adjusted class weights to mitigate the impact of class imbalance.

11.3.4 Cost-sensitive learning

Modifying the loss function of the model to incorporate the costs associated with misclassifying minority class instances encourages the model to prioritize correctly while predicting these instances.

11.3.5 Algorithmic approaches

Algorithms inherently robust to class imbalance, such as decision trees, random forests, and gradient boosting machines (GBM), are preferred choices as they can adapt decision boundaries effectively.

11.3.6 Cluster-based over-sampling

Identifying clusters within the minority class and oversampling from these clusters, rather than randomly replicating samples, can generate more meaningful synthetic instances and improve model performance.

11.3.7 Combining sampling techniques

Combining multiple sampling techniques or strategies can create a more balanced and representative training dataset, leading to improved model performance.

11.3.8 Cross-validation strategies

Utilizing stratified move-validation strategies ensures that every fold of the facts carries a consultant distribution of both minority and majority training, preventing bias in version assessment.

11.3.9 Domain-specific strategies

Tailoring the aforementioned techniques primarily based at the particular traits of the social media platform and sentiment analysis undertaking to hand ensures that the resulting models are nicely-perfect to actual-international scenarios.

By incorporating these techniques judiciously, analysts can effectively address class imbalance and develop sentiment analysis models that yield robust and reliable insights from social media data.

11.4 MODEL EVALUATION AND PERFORMANCE METRICS

Version evaluation is an essential step in the sentiment evaluation pipeline, permitting analysts to evaluate the effectiveness and reliability of their models in taking pictures and predicting sentiment from social media facts. Some other metrics, such as accuracy, F1-score, and AUC-ROC, need to be measured to analyze how well a sentiment analysis model performs. These ensure models are not only reliable but alsointerpretable [13], [24]. In this phase, we delve into various overall performance metrics and assessment techniques essential for gauging the efficacy of sentiment evaluation models:

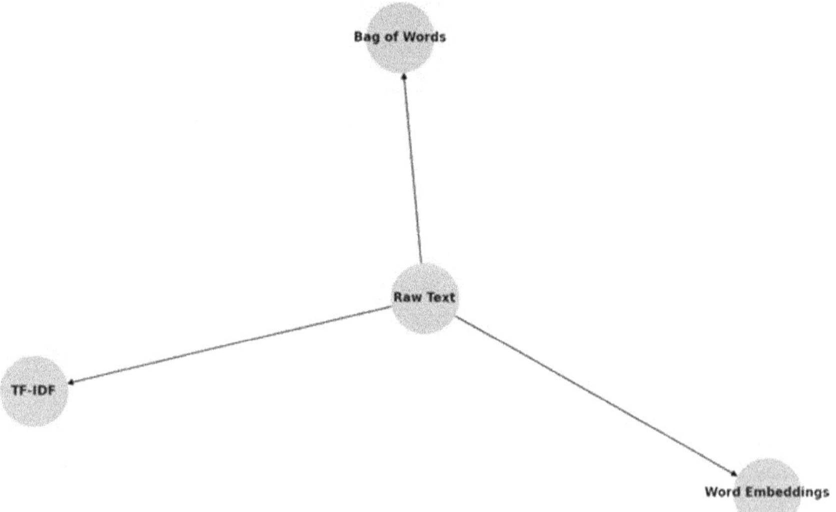

Figure 11.2 A diagram illustrating the workflow of various function engineering strategies like Bag of words, TF-IDF, and word Embeddings. this could show how raw text is converted thru every technique.

11.4.1 Confusion matrix

A confusion matrix is a desk that summarizes the overall performance of a classification model by showing the counts of genuine effective (TP), proper negative (TN), fake advantageous (FP), and fake negative (FN) predictions. Every row of the matrix represents the real magnificence, while every column represents the expected class. This matrix enables the version's conduct to be understood and areas where it is able to be making mistakes to be identified.

11.4.2 Accuracy

Accuracy is a typically used metric that measures the share of efficaciously categorized instances out of the full variety of instances. It presents a typical assessment of the version's overall performance. Mathematically, accuracy is computed because the ratio of the sum of genuine superb and authentic negative predictions to the overall wide variety of predictions:

$$Accuracy = TP + TN / TP + TN + FP + FP$$

While accuracy is intuitive and easy to understand, it may not be the most suitable metric for imbalanced datasets, where one class significantly outweighs the other(s).

11.4.3 Precision

Precision, additionally known as the wonderful predictive value, quantifies the share of real high-quality predictions amongst all tremendous predictions made by way of the model. It makes a speciality of the correctness of advantageous predictions. Mathematically, precision is computed as:

$$Precision = TP / TP + FP$$

Precision is crucial in scenarios where the cost of false positives is high, as it measures the model's ability to avoid misclassifying negative instances as positive.

11.4.4 Recall (Sensitivity)

Recall, also known as sensitivity or true positive rate, measures the proportion of true positive instances that were correctly identified by the model. It focuses on capturing all positive instances correctly. Mathematically, recall is computed as:

$$Recall = TP / TP + FN$$

Recall is vital in conditions wherein missing high quality instances (fake negatives) are extra pricey rather than incorrectly classifying negative instances as advantageous (fake positives).

11.4.5 F1-score

The F1-rating is the harmonic imply of precision and consider, imparting a balanced measure of a model's overall performance. It combines both precision and don't forget right into a single metric. Mathematically, the F1-rating is computed as:

The F1-rating reaches its satisfactory cost at 1 (best precision and keep in mind) and worst at zero. It's miles in particular are beneficial whilst the dataset is imbalanced, because it considers each false positive and false negative. Receiver operating feature (ROC) Curve:

$$F1 - Score = 2 \times (Precision \times Recall)/Precision + Recall$$

The ROC curve is a graphical illustration of the alternate-off between the proper positive price (sensitivity) and the false positive price (1 – specificity) throughout diverse threshold settings. The region below the ROC curve (AUC-ROC) is a famous metric for evaluating binary classification fashions.

11.4.6 Area Under the Precision-Recall Curve (AUC-PR)

The AUC-PR quantifies the precision-recall alternate-off by way of summarizing the version's performance throughout exclusive threshold settings. It's particularly beneficial for imbalanced datasets wherein the magnificence distribution is skewed. A higher AUC-PR shows better model overall performance in terms of both precision and this needs to be born in mind.

11.4.7 Cross-validation

Go-validation techniques, which include k-fold go-validation or stratified cross-validation, are hired to partition the dataset into a couple of subsets for education and assessment. Through iteratively educating the model on distinct subsets and comparing its overall performance on the closing data, go-validation affords greater robust estimates of version performance, lowering the risk of overfitting and making sure generalizability.

11.4.8 Domain-specific evaluation

Tailoring evaluation metrics and techniques to the specific requirements and characteristics of the social media platform and sentiment analysis task is essential for ensuring the relevance and applicability of the resulting models in real-world scenarios. This involves understanding the nuances of the target domain, such as the language used, cultural context, and prevalent sentiment expressions, and selecting evaluation metrics that align with the overarching goals of the analysis.

By employing a combination of these evaluation metrics and techniques, analysts can comprehensively assess the performance of sentiment analysis models and make informed decisions regarding model selection, fine-tuning, and deployment in real-world scenarios.

11.5 ASPECT-BASED SENTIMENT ANALYSIS

Aspect-Based Sentiment Analysis (ABSA) is a sophisticated technique within sentiment analysis that focuses on dissecting text data to discern sentiment expressed towards specific aspects, features, or entities mentioned within the text. Aspect-Based Sentiment Analysis involves identifying sentiments conveyed with regard to specific aspects or features referred to in the text. Techniques such as dependency parsing and supervised learning are useful to obtain more nuanced sentiments at the aspect level [22], [23]. In social media contexts, ABSA enables a nuanced understanding of public sentiment by identifying and analyzing opinions about various attributes of products, services, events, or topics. Let's delve deeper into the components and methodologies of ABSA:

1. Aspect Extraction Techniques:
Rule-Based Methods: These methods rely on predefined linguistic rules to identify aspects or features mentioned in the text. Rules can be based on part-of-speech tagging, syntactic patterns, or domain-specific dictionaries.

Supervised Learning Approaches: Supervised machine learning models, such as sequence labeling models (e.g., Conditional Random Fields) or neural networks (e.g., BiLSTM-CRF), can be trained on labeled data to extract aspects from text.

Unsupervised Methods: Techniques like topic modeling (e.g., Latent Dirichlet Allocation) or clustering can be employed to discover latent aspects within text data without the need for annotated training data.

2. Aspect-Based Sentiment Classification:
After extracting aspects, sentiment classification models are applied to determine the sentiment polarity (e.g., positive, negative, neutral) associated with each aspect. These models can range from traditional machine learning algorithms (e.g., SVM, Random Forest) to deep learning architectures (e.g., CNNs, Transformers).

Multi-task learning approaches, where aspect extraction and sentiment classification are jointly optimized, have shown promise in improving performance by leveraging the interdependencies between these tasks.

3. Dependency Parsing and Semantic Role Labeling:
Dependency parsing techniques analyze the grammatical structure of sentences to identify relationships between words, which can aid in associating sentiment expressions with specific aspects mentioned in the text. Semantic role labeling assigns semantic labels to words or phrases in a sentence, enabling the identification of roles such as "agent," "patient," or "theme," which can provide valuable context for sentiment analysis.

4. Aspect-Based Lexicons and Resources:
Aspect-specific sentiment lexicons contain sentiment polarity scores or sentiment phrases associated with particular aspects or domains. These lexicons serve as valuable resources for mapping sentiment expressions to relevant aspects during sentiment analysis.

5. Fine-Grained Sentiment Analysis:
Fine-grained sentiment analysis aims to capture subtle variations in sentiment expressions, such as sentiment intensity (e.g., strong positive vs. weak positive) or sentiment modifiers (e.g., very positive vs. slightly positive), within each aspect.

6. Cross-Domain and Transfer Learning:
Cross-domain ABSA involves adapting sentiment analysis models trained on one domain to perform sentiment analysis in another domain. Transfer learning techniques, such as pre-training on large-scale datasets or domain-specific feature engineering, can facilitate knowledge transfer between domains.

7. Evaluation and Metrics:
Evaluation metrics for ABSA encompass aspect-level metrics (e.g., aspect extraction accuracy, aspect-level precision, recall, and F1-score) and sentiment classification metrics (e.g., accuracy, precision, recall, F1-score, aspect-level sentiment consistency). These metrics provide insights into the performance of ABSA systems.

8. Toolkits and Frameworks:
Various toolkits and frameworks, such as ABSA Toolkits (ABSAT), Stanford CoreNLP, or spaCy, offer functionalities for aspect extraction, sentiment classification, dependency parsing, and other ABSA-related tasks, streamlining the development of ABSA systems.

By leveraging these methodologies and techniques, analysts can extract nuanced sentiment insights from social media data, enabling organizations to make informed decisions based on a comprehensive understanding of public opinion towards specific aspects or entities of interest. ABSA finds applications across diverse domains, including product reviews, customer feedback analysis, brand monitoring, market research, and beyond.

11.6 REAL-TIME SENTIMENT ANALYSIS

Real-time sentiment analysis is a dynamic process that involves continuously monitoring and analyzing incoming streams of data, such as social media posts, customer reviews, or news articles, to extract and understand sentiment as it unfolds. Real-time sentiment analysis frameworks, such as Apache Kafka, allow organizations to continuously track customer sentiment and respond accordingly to the emerging trend [24]. This has had applications in various sectors like retail, healthcare, and financial services.

In this section, we explore the techniques, tools, and considerations involved in implementing real-time sentiment analysis systems:

11.6.1 Streaming data sources

Real-time sentiment analysis systems typically ingest data from streaming sources such as social media APIs (e.g., Twitter Streaming API), news feeds, online forums, or customer review platforms. These sources provide a constant flow of data for analysis.

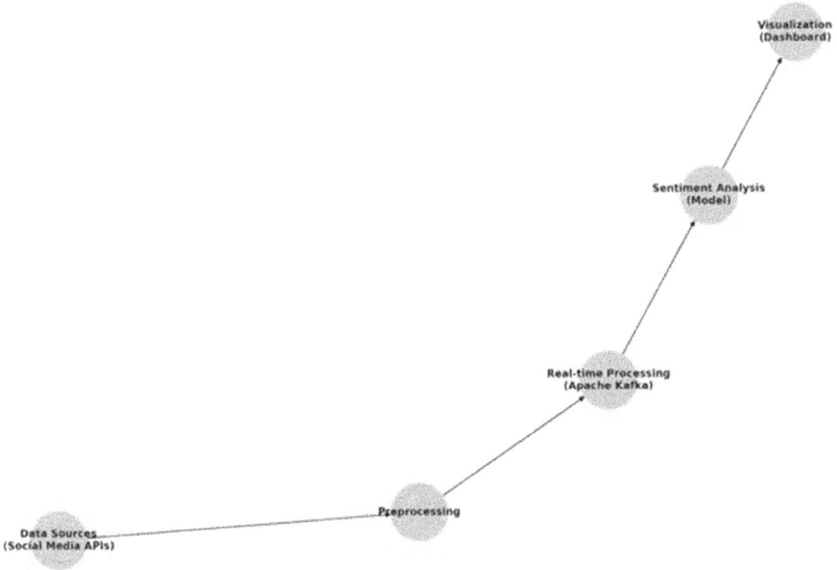

Figure 11.3 An architecture diagram of a real-time sentiment analysis system. This could include data sources (social media APIs), preprocessing steps, real-time processing frameworks (like Apache Kafka), and visualization tools.

11.6.2 Data preprocessing

Preprocessing techniques such as tokenization, normalization, and filtering are applied to incoming data streams to prepare them for sentiment analysis. This ensures that the text data is clean and formatted consistently before sentiment analysis algorithms are applied.

11.6.3 Real-time sentiment analysis algorithms

Various algorithms can be used for real-time sentiment analysis, including lexicon-based methods, machine learning models (e.g., Support Vector Machines, Naive Bayes), and deep learning architectures (e.g., Recurrent Neural Networks, Transformers). These algorithms analyze text data to classify sentiment in real-time.

11.6.4 Scalable processing architecture

Real-time sentiment analysis systems require scalable processing architectures capable of handling high volumes of incoming data streams efficiently. Technologies such as Apache Kafka, Apache Storm, Apache Flink, or AWS Kinesis provide scalable, distributed processing capabilities for real-time data analysis.

11.6.5 Streaming analytics platforms

Streaming analytics platforms like Apache Spark Streaming, Apache Beam, or Apache Samza offer frameworks for building real-time sentiment analysis pipelines. These platforms provide libraries and APIs for data processing, machine learning, and streaming analytics.

11.6.6 Feature engineering and model deployment

Feature engineering techniques, such as TF-IDF (Term Frequency-Inverse Document Frequency) or word embeddings, may be applied to extract relevant features from text data for sentiment analysis. Trained sentiment analysis models are deployed within the real-time processing pipeline to classify sentiment in incoming data streams.

11.6.7 Real-time visualization and monitoring

Real-time sentiment analysis systems often include visualization dashboards and monitoring tools to track sentiment trends, visualize sentiment distributions, and identify emerging topics or events. Visualization techniques such as word clouds, sentiment heatmaps, or time-series plots are commonly used for real-time monitoring.

11.6.8 Latency and throughput optimization

Optimizing latency and throughput is crucial for real-time sentiment analysis systems to ensure timely processing of incoming data streams. Techniques such as parallel processing, distributed computing, and efficient resource allocation help minimize processing delays and handle spikes in data volume.

11.6.9 Feedback loop and model updating

Real-time sentiment analysis systems may incorporate feedback loops to continuously improve model performance. User feedback or labeled data from human annotators can be used to retrain sentiment analysis models periodically and adapt to evolving language patterns and sentiment expressions.

11.6.10 Ethical and privacy considerations

Ethical considerations, such as data privacy, consent, and bias mitigation, are paramount in real-time sentiment analysis systems. Organizations must ensure compliance with regulations and ethical guidelines while handling sensitive user data and analyzing sentiment in real-time. The sentiment analysis also poses ethical concerns such as bias mitigation, data privacy, and transparency. The previous studies suggest the need for fair-aware models and strong privacy frameworks to ensure responsible use of sentiment analysis systems [12], [20].

By incorporating these techniques and considerations, organizations can develop robust real-time sentiment analysis systems capable of extracting actionable insights from streaming data sources and staying abreast of public opinion and sentiment as it evolves in real-time.

11.7 REAL WORLD CASE STUDIES AND EXAMPLES

For this purpose, in the following and the final section of this chapter, we will demonstrate the real-life applications of the concepts of sentiment analysis from different fields. Consequently, the present work provides a comprehension of how they were categorized, how communication sentiment analysis can be designed and utilized for various tasks and issues to yield outcomes.

Case Study 1: Retail Industry
An online firm navigating for product selling collected opinions through the site aiming to employ sentiment analysis. Similarly, the retailer of the products may look at reviews and mentions on social media to also note the challenges that customers are facing. For example, a high level of negativity was in options such as shipping's delay and issues concerning product

quality. As for the potential benefits, which arose, if going deep into detail, such as analyzing the reviews, the retailer would be able to determine, which aspect of the logistics and quality maintenance was lackluster.

As the shipping time was an issue the retailer aimed at enhancing its functional competence in operation by working with different and more competent courier service providers together with addressing the issues related to the supply chain that resulted from long shipment periods and stockout. This change has not only occurred with the added advantage of increase in delivery time, but it also has eliminated a number of complaints that were made because of delayed deliveries as well. It also settled with several clients for product defects that were a major concern causing immense losses to its clients, and in response, the retailer committed to a relatively enhanced quality management program that seeks to detect the weakness in products before delivering them to consumers.

The results were significant: With the help of 'customer' evaluation results, the number increased by 15 percentage points in six months; 'customer' loyalty was also improved as well as a number of positive comments marked as 'word of mouth' on the internet. As such, this case enables the demonstration of how sentiment analysis provides the data used at the operational level and the resultant enhancement of services and customer retention.

Case Study 2: Financial Services

A particular large financial institution used real-time sentiment analysis to measure consumers' reception of its new mobile application for banking. They could escalate complaints that are pointed in the social platform by users, and by combining sentiment analysis with their customer service platform. It also made it easier for the institution to regulate feedback collection on a real-time basis and attend to concerns which were more important.

Concerning the overall sentiment analysis which is shown in the table below, users were especially disappointed in the app's navigational options, and slight issues with the performance. The financial institution's development team responded by rapidly releasing updates that address the usability and other issues. Furthermore, the customer service was offering help in specific cases to unhappy clients and actively collecting more detailed feedback.

While it improved customers' satisfaction due to anticipating their needs, it decreased the number of support tickets by 20%. The institution also stated that on S. and the app store, responses typical of satisfied customers could be seen, such as complimenting fast responses and improvements. The above case illustrates that when it comes to dealing with customers' impressions real-time monitoring of sentiments is crucial for positive impacts on products.

Case Study 3: Healthcare
In the context of the healthcare sector, the application of sentiment analysis was used to analyze patients' feedback on the services offered by hospitals. Thus, the result of such analysis could provide answers to questions about the priorities of which aspects should be paid attention at the hospitals: waiting time, staff behavior, or even the condition of the facilities.

A specific hospital identified that numerous complaints addressed long waiting times in the emergency department and perceived rudeness of staff. To mitigate these challenges, the following changes were made by the hospital; change in staff working time, to cover most of the shift periods in a day, and the training for customer service and patient handling.

From the results of these findings, measures were made to integrate modifications and yield better reactions from the patients and lower patient attrition rates. Health review sites also rated the hospital better and this has assisted in drawing more clientele for the hospital. This chapter demonstrates how sentiment analysis can be used in the healthcare industry regarding patient outcomes and health organization's performance.

Case Study 4: Hospitality
An example from a large hotel chain was the use of sentiment analysis to the company's guests and therefore increase the quality of service delivery. The results collected from the hotel chain stemmed from the review platforms of travel sites and social media to comprehend the guest satisfaction or dissatisfaction index in certain concerns. Cleanliness, noise and check-in/check-out were the most frequent topics in the negative feedback.

As a response, the hotel chain began the following activities to come up with a solution. They raised the pressure and the frequency of room cleaning to make the rooms cleaner, improved sound isolation in rooms to meet guests' complaints about sounds coming from other rooms, and finally, they also improved the check-in and check-out process due to enhanced staff training and better technologies.

Therefore, within three months, the hotel chain achieved an increment in positive feedback by 10% and a measurable turnover in guest loyalty in the chain. They also reported a higher level of satisfaction during the post-stay feedback endeavors as a result of the specific areas of enhancement based on sentiment analysis.

Case Study 5: Telecommunications
A group of managers of a large telecommunications company employed a sentiment analysis to identify customers' attitudes towards their customer service and products. Looking at the call center transcripts, posts on social media and reviews of the company, the firm would establish that some of the common complaints include network reliability, billing issues, and quality of customer service.

The study showed that the analysis of sentiment conformed to the customer's complaints with the network reliability as being the most important factor of concern, seconded by dissatisfaction with the billing process and customer responses. The specific area addressed is expansion of network facilities to minimize disruptions and enhance the company's performance. They also reformulated the manner in which they bill their customers to make their charges clearer than before while offering the customer service personnel extra training to enhance their ability to solve issues and the quality of their social dealings.

These changes helped to transform the customer relations significantly, and the number of complaints was decreased; meanwhile, the satisfaction level of the next year was increased by 25%. The company also experienced a decrease in the churn rates whereby customers remained with the company due to the enhanced quality services. The following case study will depict how sentiment analysis techniques are quite instrumental in coping with some of the vital operational challenges and in overall customer satisfaction in the telecom sector.

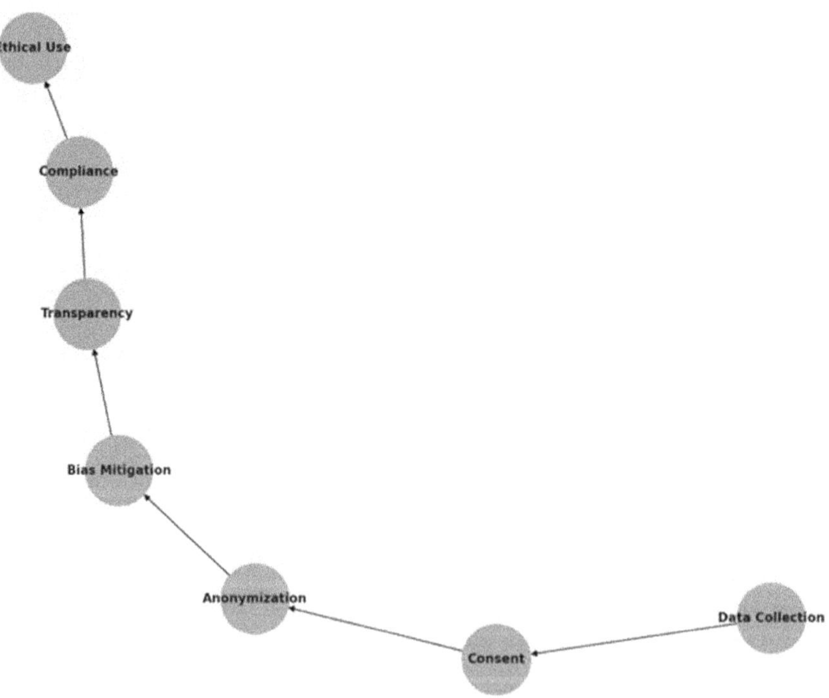

Figure 11.4 A flowchart or checklist of ethical considerations and steps to ensure data privacy and bias mitigation in sentiment analysis projects.

Such examples are illustrative of particular spheres where sentiment analysis can be applied and they may be invaluable if the outcomes demonstrating higher efficacy have to be provided to address alterations and developments in various contexts. Therefore, the result of sentiment analysis is useful for CEOs and managers regardless of the type of business because it helps to draw an idea of customer opinions about the company, its weaknesses, and, therefore, create the corresponding effective long-term strategies for increasing the level of customer satisfaction and loyalty. Considering the vast opportunities that SA offers in terms of flexibility and effectiveness of its use, it can be considered among the key solutions existing in today's world, which would enable organizations to sustain their competitive advantage and be ready to meet demand for and customer preferences.

11.8 FUTURE PROOFING SENTIMENT ANALYSIS TECHNIQUES

Given the continual expansion and evolution of social media platforms and Sentiment Analysis techniques, it should be borne in mind that the tools to use and the methods employed in this chapter might attain Web obsolescence pretty soon. A continually learning party will thus be on the edge to stay relevant in this regard. Researchers and practitioners shall be up-to-date in up-and-coming trends in NLP, ML, and data analytics for the continued effectiveness of their sentiment analysis systems.

11.8.1 Keeping up with technological advancements

The field of NLP and ML is highly dynamic, and new models, algorithms, and frameworks keep pouring in. In future-proofing techniques for sentiment analysis, one should:

1. Monitor Academic Research: The papers to be found in leading conferences and journals like ACL, EMNLP, and NeurIPS should be looked over regularly.
2. Adopt State-of-the-Art Models: Use the latest models of NLP. Transformer-based models like BERT, GPT, T5 have appeared quite successful in the comprehension of context and nuances in text so far. Keep yourself updated with Model advancement and integrate the new model, and it will increase the accuracy of Sentiment Analysis many folds.
3. Leverage Open-Source Tools: Use and contribute to open-source libraries and projects. Open-source tools, such as TensorFlow, PyTorch, Hugging Face's Transformers, and spaCy, for example, will have the community updating them; hence, one will get access to all the latest development.

4. Invest in Continuous Learning: Constantly provide education and training for data scientists and engineers. Online courses, workshops, and certifications can keep teams constantly updated with new techniques/tools.

11.8.2 Enhancing data collection and processing

As social media systems and communication channels evolve, the assets and codecs of information will diversify. To hold robust sentiment analysis competencies:

1. Expand Data Sources: Incorporate records from emerging social media platforms, forums, and different virtual verbal exchange channels. This ensures a comprehensive knowledge of sentiment throughout extraordinary person bases and contexts.
2. Real-Time Data Processing: Implement real-time data collection and processing pipelines to deal with the consistent glide of data from diverse platforms. This is crucial for well-timed and relevant sentiment evaluation, particularly in industries wherein rapid response is important.
3. Advanced Preprocessing Techniques: Develop state-of-the-art facts preprocessing methods to address noise, slang, emojis, and other casual language factors commonplace in social media texts. Techniques along with tokenization, normalization, and contextual embedding are crucial for accurately decoding sentiment.

11.8.3 Emphasizing ethical considerations and bias mitigation

Ethical considerations and bias mitigation are an increasing number within sentiment analysis. Ensuring that sentiment evaluation structures are fair, obvious, and unbiased involves:

1. Bias Detection and Correction: Regularly audit sentiment analysis fashions for biases associated with race, gender, age, and other demographics. Use strategies including fairness-conscious ML to pick out and mitigate biases.
2. Transparency and Explainability: Strive for transparency in sentiment analysis methodologies. Use explainable AI (XAI) techniques to make model decisions comprehensible to stakeholders and end-users, fostering consideration in the machine.
3. Privacy and Data Security: Implement robust information privacy and safety features to shield user records. Adhere to regulations consisting of GDPR and CCPA, ensuring that sentiment evaluation

practices appreciate consumer privateness and comply with felony standards.

11.8.4 Integration with broader systems

Sentiment analysis does not perform in isolation. Integrating sentiment evaluation with broader AI structures can increase its impact:

1. Multimodal Sentiment Analysis: Combine text analysis with different facts sorts including pix, films, and audio for a richer know-how of sentiment. Techniques like visible sentiment analysis and speech sentiment evaluation can offer deeper insights.
2. Interdisciplinary Approaches: Collaborate with experts in psychology, sociology, and linguistics to decorate the interpretative electricity of sentiment analysis models. This interdisciplinary technique can assist in discovering deeper emotional and cognitive dimensions of sentiment.

Three. Feedback Loops and Model Updating: Establish comments loops wherein version predictions are continuously verified and subtle based on real-global outcomes. This iterative procedure ensures that sentiment evaluation models continue to be correct and relevant over time.

11.8.5 Case studies on adaptation and innovation

11.8.5.1 Case study 1: adapting to new social media platforms

An era agency centered on social media analytics observed an enormous shift in consumer engagement from traditional structures like Facebook and Twitter to more modern ones inclusive of TikTok and Clubhouse. To adapt, the organization expanded its statistics collection abilities to include those platforms, developing custom APIs and scraping equipment to acquire data. They also update their sentiment evaluation fashions to handle the specific codecs of those systems, together with short video transcripts and audio snippets. This edition allowed the company to provide correct sentiment insights to clients inquisitive about these emerging markets.

11.8.5.2 Case study 2: leveraging advanced NLP techniques

A monetary offerings organization sought to beautify its sentiment analysis abilities to better recognize market sentiment and expect inventory moves. By integrating transformer-primarily based fashions like BERT and GPT-3, the company advanced the accuracy of their sentiment predictions. They additionally hired first-class tuning strategies that use area-particular facts to tailor the fashions to financial texts, ensuing in extra specific sentiment insights that considerably improve their buying and selling strategies.

11.8.5.3 Case study 3: implementing bias mitigation

A healthcare employer used sentiment analysis to gauge patient delight and remarks. After identifying biases in their initial fashions that disproportionately favored comments from more youthful patients, the organization applied equity-conscious ML strategies to mitigate these biases. They adjusted their training facts and algorithms to make certain a more balanced illustration of all patient demographics, leading to greater equitable and accurate sentiment analysis consequences.

The destiny-proofing of sentiment analysis strategies entails continuous version and learning. By staying abreast of technological improvements, expanding information assets, emphasizing ethical issues, integrating with broader AI systems, and learning from adaptive case studies, researchers and practitioners can make certain the sustained effectiveness and relevance of sentiment evaluation. This proactive approach will allow agencies to keep a competitive aspect and preserve deriving valuable insights from sentiment information.

11.9 ETHICAL CONSIDERATION

Ethical considerations are vital to each element of sentiment analysis, especially while dealing with social media facts. The cornerstone of moral sentiment analysis lies in ensuring information privacy and obtaining informed consent from customers whose information is being analyzed. This includes adhering to relevant facts, safety regulations, and clearly communicating the motive and implications of sentiment analysis to users. Transparency and explainability are similarly crucial, as customers, stakeholders, and affected parties should understand how sentiment evaluation is conducted, together with the algorithms used and any potential biases or limitations. Bias mitigation strategies are crucial to prevent unfair or discriminatory consequences, necessitating thorough checks and ongoing tracking of model performance. Accountability frameworks help make sure that individuals and organizations are held responsible for the moral implications of sentiment evaluation sports. Moreover, accountable use of sentiment evaluation outcomes entails thinking about the wider societal impact and potential consequences of evaluation findings. Researchers and practitioners ought to prioritize moral ideas all through the sentiment evaluation manner, from records series to interpretation and application of effects. This consists of promoting variety and inclusivity in studies and practice to address capability biases and ensure equitable results for all people. By integrating ethical issues into every degree of sentiment evaluation, stakeholders can construct, agree with, uphold integrity, and make a contribution to tremendous societal effects even by respecting the rights and privacy of individuals involved.

11.10 ADVANTAGES, DISADVANTAGES OF SENTIMENT ANALYSIS

11.10.1 Advantages

Sentiment analysis gives a large number of benefits across numerous domain names, making it an effective device for knowledge of public opinion, client sentiment, and market traits. Here are some key advantages highlighted in an e-book chapter:

1. Insight Generation: Sentiment analysis permits agencies to advantage precious insights into patron reviews, alternatives, and attitudes in the direction of products, offerings, or manufacturers. By studying large volumes of textual facts from sources like social media, opinions, and surveys, businesses can pick out rising traits, sentiments, and regions for development.

2. Customer Engagement: Understanding client sentiment in real-time permits businesses to have interactions with their audience more effectively. By right away addressing issues, responding to comments, and leveraging nice sentiment, corporations can decorate client satisfaction, loyalty, and brand reputation.

3. Market Intelligence: Sentiment analysis gives precious marketplace intelligence by way of monitoring customer sentiment closer to competition, industry traits, and market traits. This record permits corporations to make informed selections concerning product development, advertising and marketing strategies, and competitive positioning.

4. Risk Management: Sentiment evaluation helps organizations pick out and mitigate ability risks, together with negative publicity, customer dissatisfaction, or reputational harm. By monitoring sentiment throughout various channels, corporations can proactively address troubles earlier before they deteriorate into crises.

5. Product Development: Sentiment analysis aids in product development by amassing remarks on present products or services and identifying areas for enhancement or innovation. By studying consumer sentiment, groups can tailor their services to meet evolving client alternatives and marketplace needs.

6. Brand Monitoring: Sentiment evaluation lets organizations reveal brand sentiment and tune how their logo is perceived with the aid of the public. By monitoring social media conversations, reviews,

and mentions, businesses can gauge emblem sentiment, pick out influencers, and determine the effectiveness of branding techniques.

7. Campaign Evaluation: Sentiment evaluation helps compare the effectiveness of advertising campaigns, ad campaigns, and promotional sports. By analyzing sentiment earlier, at some point of, and after campaigns, agencies can determine their effect on client sentiment, emblem belief, and buy purpose.

8. Opinion Mining: Sentiment analysis allows opinion mining by using mechanically extracting and summarizing evaluations, sentiments, and viewpoints from huge volumes of textual records. This enables companies to gain complete insight into public opinion on numerous subjects, issues, or occasions.

9. Predictive Analytics: Sentiment evaluation may be used for predictive analytics, forecasting future tendencies, patron conduct, and market dynamics based totally on historic sentiment facts. By studying styles and traits in sentiment, businesses can assume marketplace shifts, customer preferences, and rising possibilities.

10. Cost and Time Efficiency: Sentiment analysis automates the system of analyzing textual data, saving organizations time and resources as compared to manual analysis. By getting to know algorithms and herbal language processing strategies, organizations can efficiently method big volumes of information and extract actionable insights at scale.

11.10.2 Disadvantages

While sentiment evaluation offers many blessings, it also comes with certain boundaries and demanding situations that need to be taken into consideration. Here are some of the negative aspects of sentiment evaluation:

1. Subjectivity and Ambiguity: Sentiment analysis often deals with subjective and ambiguous language, making it hard to appropriately interpret sentiment. Sarcasm, irony, slang, and cultural nuances can result in misclassification of sentiment, lowering the reliability of evaluation outcomes.

2. Contextual Understanding: Sentiment evaluation algorithms may additionally struggle to comprehend the context in which sentiment is expressed, leading to misinterpretation of sentiment. Understanding context is critical for accurately shooting the intended meaning behind text, specially in complicated or nuanced conditions.

3. Language Complexity: Sentiment evaluation becomes extra hard when handling multilingual or code-switching texts. Differences in

grammar, syntax, and cultural norms throughout languages can affect the overall performance of sentiment analysis models, requiring variation and customization for each language.

4. Imbalanced Datasets: Imbalanced datasets, in which one sentiment elegance dominates over others, can bias sentiment evaluation effects and reduce the accuracy of fashions, especially for minority classes. Addressing elegance imbalance requires careful facts preprocessing and model optimization techniques.

5. Domain Specificity: Sentiment evaluation fashions skilled on one area won't generalize well to other domains due to differences in language use, sentiment expressions, and topic relevance. Domain variation strategies are hard to customize sentiment evaluation fashions for unique domains and make certain accurate results.

6. Noise and Irrelevant Information: Social media records frequently carry noise, beside the point records, and junk mail, that could intrude with sentiment evaluation and bring misguided outcomes. Preprocessing strategies are required to filter noise and ensure that sentiment evaluation models consciousness on applicable content material.

7. Ethical and Privacy Concerns: Sentiment analysis raises moral concerns associated with privacy, consent, and information usage, particularly whilst reading person-generated content material from social media structures. Respecting consumer privacy, acquiring knowledgeable consent, and adhering to ethical recommendations are essential for accomplishing sentiment analysis ethically.

8. Over Reliance on Text Data: Sentiment analysis relies heavily on textual information, which may not continually capture the total spectrum of human emotions and sentiments. Integrating different modalities such as snapshots, motion pictures, or audio should provide richer context and improve the accuracy of sentiment evaluation consequences.

9. Bias and Fairness Issues: Sentiment analysis models can also show off biases, reflecting the biases gift within the training facts or the underlying algorithms. Biased fashions can lead to unfair or discriminatory results, highlighting the importance of bias detection, mitigation, and equity-aware version improvement.

10. Limitations of Automated Systems: Automated sentiment analysis structures might also lack the nuanced knowledge and interpretive skills of human analysts, mainly due to errors or misinterpretations in sentiment categories. Human oversight and validation are often necessary to ensure the reliability and accuracy of sentiment analysis effects.

11.11 CONCLUSION

In conclusion, sentiment evaluation stands as a powerful tool for extracting precious insights from textual records, mainly inside the context of social media. Through the software of natural language processing techniques and machine-gaining knowledge of algorithms, sentiment evaluation permits businesses, companies, and researchers to apprehend public opinion, client sentiment, marketplace traits, and rising topics in real-time. By studying sentiment throughout numerous channels, which includes social media posts, client critiques, information articles, and surveys, stakeholders could make knowledgeable decisions, beautify client experiences, and force enterprise boom. However, while sentiment analysis gives numerous blessings, it also comes with inherent limitations and challenges. Issues which include subjectivity, ambiguity, language complexity, and bias require careful consideration and mitigation to make certain the reliability and accuracy of sentiment evaluation outcomes. Moreover, moral worries related to data privacy, consent, equity, and bias ought to be addressed to behavior sentiment evaluation ethically and responsibly. Despite these challenges, the capacity benefits of sentiment analysis are great, ranging from market intelligence and logo tracking to customer engagement and threat control. By leveraging sentiment evaluation efficiently and ethically, corporations can have an aggressive edge, build consideration with stakeholders, and force tremendous social impact. Moving forward, enduring improvements in sentiment analysis strategies, coupled with a dedication to ethical practice, will in addition beautify the application and reliability of sentiment evaluation in a rapidly evolving digital panorama.

REFERENCES

1. Tammina, Srikanth. "A hybrid learning approach for sentiment classification in Telugu language." *2020 International Conference on Artificial Intelligence and Signal Processing (AISP)*. IEEE, (2020).
2. Karageorgou, Ioanna, Panagiotis Liakos, and Alex Delis. "A Sentiment Analysis Service Platform for Streamed Multilingual Tweets." *2020 IEEE International Conference on Big Data (Big Data)*. IEEE, (2020).
3. Antonakaki, Despoina, Paraskevi Fragopoulou, and Sotiris Ioannidis. "A survey of Twitter research: Data model, graph structure, sentiment analysis and attacks." *Expert Systems with Applications* 164 (2021): 114006.
4. Shanmugavadivel, Kogilavani, et al. "An analysis of machine learning models for sentiment analysis of Tamil code-mixed data." *Computer Speech & Language* 76 (2022): 101407.
5. Raviya, K., and Mary Vennila. "An implementation of hybrid enhanced sentiment analysis system using Spark ML Pipeline: A big data analytics framework." *International Journal of Advanced Computer Science and Applications* 12.5 (2021): 323–329.

6. Anbukkarasi, S., and S. Varadhaganapathy. "Analyzing sentiment in Tamil tweets using deep neural network." *2020 Fourth International Conference on Computing Methodologies and Communication (ICCMC)*. IEEE, (2020).

7. Chakravarthi, Bharathi Raja, et al. "Dravidiancodemix: Sentiment analysis and offensive language identification dataset for Dravidian languages in code-mixed text." *Language Resources and Evaluation* 56.3 (2022): 765–806.

8. Kannan, R. Ramesh, Ratnavel Rajalakshmi, and Lokesh Kumar. "IndicBERT based approach for sentiment analysis on code-mixed Tamil Tweets." In *FIRE (Working Notes)* (pp. 729–736). (2021).

9. Ahamed, M. R., and S. P. Arachchi. "LSTM Based Emotion Analysis of Text in Tamil Language." 7th International Conference on Advances in Technology and Computing (ICATC 2022), (pp. 73–79). Publisher Faculty of Computing and Technology, University of Kelaniya Sri Lanka, (2022).

10. Sujatha, E., and R. Radha. "New Education Policy 2020: A sentiment classification." *Indian Journal of Science and Technology* 16.9 (2023): 614–621.

11. Se, Shriya, et al. "Predicting the sentimental reviews in Tamil movies using machine learning algorithms." *Indian Journal of Science and Technology* 9.45 (2016): 1–5.

12. Ahmad, Gazi Imtiyaz, Jimmy Singla, and Nikita Nikita. "Review on sentiment analysis of Indian languages with a special focus on code mixed Indian languages." *2019 International Conference on Automation, Computational and Technology Management (ICACTM)*. IEEE, (2019).

13. Bhuvan, Malladihalli S., et al. "Semantic sentiment analysis using context specific grammar." *International Conference on Computing, Communication & Automation*. IEEE, (2015).

14. Ramanathan, Vallikannu, T. Meyyappan, and S. M. Thamarai. "Sentiment analysis: an approach for analyzing Tamil movie reviews using Tamil tweets." *Recent Advances in Mathematical Research and Computer Science* 3 (2021): 28–39.

15. Edara, Deepak Chowdary, et al. "Sentiment analysis and text categorization of cancer medical records with LSTM." *Journal of Ambient Intelligence and Humanized Computing* 14.5 (2023): 5309–5325.

16. Jha, Bineet Kumar, G. G. Sivasankari, and K. R. Venugopal. "Sentiment analysis for E-commerce products using natural language processing." *Annals of the Romanian Society for Cell Biology* (2021): 166–175.

17. Ramesh Babu, Suba Sri. Sentiment analysis in Tamil language using hybrid deep learning approach. Diss. Dublin, National College of Ireland, (2022).

18. Thavareesan, Sajeetha, and Sinnathamby Mahesan. "Sentiment analysis in Tamil texts: A study on machine learning techniques and feature representation." *2019 14th Conference on Industrial and Information Systems (ICIIS)*. IEEE, (2019).

19. Shalini, K., et al. "Sentiment analysis of Indian languages using convolutional neural networks." *2018 International Conference on Computer Communication and Informatics (ICCCI)*. IEEE, (2018).

20. Soumya, S., and K. V. Pramod. "Sentiment analysis of malayalam tweets using machine learning techniques." *ICT Express* 6.4 (2020): 300–305.

21. Padmamala, R., and V. Prema. "Sentiment analysis of online Tamil contents using recursive neural network models approach for Tamil language." *2017 IEEE International Conference on Smart Technologies and Management for Computing, Communication, Controls, Energy and Materials (ICSTM)*. IEEE, (2017).

22. Phani, Shanta, Shibamouli Lahiri, and Arindam Biswas. "Sentiment analysis of tweets in three Indian languages." *Proceedings of the 6th Workshop on South and Southeast Asian Natural Language Processing (WSSANLP2016)*. The COLING 2016 Organizing Committee, (2016).

23. Sharmista, A., and M. Ramaswami. "Sentiment analysis on Tamil reviews as products in social media using machine learning techniques: A Novel Study." *Madurai Kamaraj University Madurai-625* 21 (2020).

24. Jacob, Sharon Susan, and R. Vijayakumar. "Sentiment analysis over Twitter Bigdata using modified meanshift clustering algorithm." *Journal of Critical Reviews* 7.15 (2020): 5835–5841.

Index

For Product Safety Concerns and Information please contact our EU
representative GPSR@taylorandfrancis.com
Taylor & Francis Verlag GmbH, Kaufingerstraße 24, 80331 München, Germany